T0226888

Disparities and Determinants of Health in Surgical Oncology

Editor

OLUWADAMILOLA M. FAYANJU

SURGICAL ONCOLOGY CLINICS OF NORTH AMERICA

www.surgonc.theclinics.com

Consulting Editor
TIMOTHY M. PAWLIK

January 2022 • Volume 31 • Number 1

ELSEVIER

1600 John F. Kennedy Boulevard • Suite 1800 • Philadelphia, Pennsylvania, 19103-2899

http://www.theclinics.com

SURGICAL ONCOLOGY CLINICS OF NORTH AMERICA Volume 31, Number 1
January 2022 ISSN 1055-3207, ISBN-13: 978-0-323-84914-2

Editor: John Vassallo (j.vassallo@elsevier.com)
Developmental Editor: Diana Ang

Surgical Oncology Clinics of North America (ISSN 1055-3207) is published quarterly by Elsevier Inc., 360 Park Avenue South, New York, NY 10010-1710. Months of publication are January, April, July, and October. Business and Editorial Offices: 1600 John F. Kennedy Blvd., Ste. 1800, Philadelphia, PA 19103-2899. Customer Service Office: 3251 Riverport Lane, Maryland Heights, MO 63043. Periodicals postage paid at New York, NY and additional mailing offices. Subscription prices are $325.00 per year (US individuals), $776.00 (US institutions) $100.00 (US student/resident), $363.00 (Canadian individuals), $803.00 (Canadian institutions), $100.00 (Canadian student/resident), $470.00 (foreign individuals), $803.00 (foreign institutions), and $205.00 (foreign student/resident). Foreign air speed delivery is included in all *Clinics* subscription prices. All prices are subject to change without notice. **POSTMASTER**: Send address changes to *Surgical Oncology Clinics of North America,* Elsevier Health Science Division, Subscription Customer Service, 3251 Riverport Lane, Maryland Heights, MO 63043. **Customer Service: 1-800-654-2452 (US and Canada). 314-447-8871 (outside US and Canada). Fax: 314-447-8029. E-mail: journalscustomerservice-usa@elsevier.com (for print support); journalsonline support-usa@elsevier.com (for online support).**

Reprints. For copies of 100 or more, of articles in this publication, please contact the Commercial Reprints Department, Elsevier Inc., 360 Park Avenue South, New York, New York 10010-1710. Tel. 212-633-3874; Fax: 212-633-3820; E-mail: reprints@elsevier.com.

Surgical Oncology Clinics of North America is covered in *MEDLINE/PubMed (Index Medicus)* and *EMBASE/ Excerpta Medica, Current Contents/Clinical Medicine,* and *ISI/BIOMED.*

Contributors

CONSULTING EDITOR

TIMOTHY M. PAWLIK, MD, MPH, PhD, FACS, FRACS (Hon.)
Professor and Chair, Department of Surgery, The Urban Meyer III and Shelley Meyer Chair for Cancer Research, Professor of Surgery, Oncology, Health Services Management and Policy, Surgeon in Chief, The Ohio State University Wexner Medical Center, Columbus, Ohio

EDITOR

OLUWADAMILOLA M. FAYANJU, MD, MA, MPHS, FACS
The Helen O. Dickens Presidential Associate Professor and Chief of Breast Surgery, Department of Surgery; Surgical Director, Rena Rowan Breast Center, Abramson Cancer Center, Perelman School of Medicine at the University of Pennsylvania, Penn Medicine, Philadelphia, Pennsylvania

AUTHORS

FOLUSO O. ADEMUYIWA, MD, MPH, MSCI
Associate Professor of Medicine, Department of Medicine, Washington University School of Medicine, St Louis, Missouri

MEGAN BARRETT, MD
Assistant Professor, Department of Obstetrics and Gynecology, Duke University Medical Center, Durham, North Carolina

CALLISIA N. CLARKE, MD, MS
Assistant Professor of Surgery, Division of Surgical Oncology, Milwaukee, Wisconsin

JACQUELYN DILLON, MS
Department of Surgery, Duke University Medical Center, Durham, North Carolina

MATTHEW E.B. DIXON, MD, FACS
Assistant Professor of Surgery, Division of Surgical Oncology, Penn State Health Milton S. Hershey Medical Center, Hershey, Pennsylvania

VISHNUKAMAL GOLLA, MD, MPH
Duke National Clinician Scholars Program, Department of Surgery, Division of Urology, Duke University Medical Center, Duke Cancer Institute, Duke-Margolis Policy Center, Durham Veterans Affairs Health Care System, Durham, North Carolina

RACHEL A. GREENUP, MD, MPH
Division of Surgical Oncology, Department of Surgery, Yale School of Medicine, The Breast Center at Smilow Cancer Hospital at Yale New Haven, New Haven, Connecticut

NIRAJ J. GUSANI, MD, MS, FACS
Chief, Section of Surgical Oncology, Baptist MD Anderson Cancer Center, Jacksonville, Florida

SCARLETT HAO, MD
Resident Physician, Department of Surgery, Brody School of Medicine at East Carolina University, Greenville, North Carolina

KEVIN S. HUGHES, MD
Professor of Surgery, Surgical Oncology, Massachusetts General Hospital, Boston, Massachusetts

GABRIEL D. IVEY, MD
Fellow, Complex General Surgical Oncology, Department of Surgery, Division of Surgical Oncology, The Johns Hopkins University, Baltimore, Maryland

FABIAN M. JOHNSTON, MD, MHS
Associate Professor of Surgery and Oncology, Chief, Division of Gastrointestinal Surgical Oncology, Director, Peritoneal Surface Malignancy Program, Program Director, Complex General Surgical Oncology Fellowship, Department of Surgery, Division of Surgical Oncology, The Johns Hopkins University, Baltimore, Maryland

DEBORAH R. KAYE, MD, MS
Assistant Professor, Department of Surgery, Division of Urology, Duke University Medical Center, Duke Cancer Institute, Duke-Margolis Policy Center, Durham, North Carolina

UGWUJI N. MADUEKWE, MD, MMSc, MPH
Assistant Professor of Surgery, Division of Surgical Oncology and Endocrine Surgery, Department of Surgery, The University of North Carolina at Chapel Hill, Chapel Hill, North Carolina

KATHLEEN MARULANDA, MD, MS
General Surgery Resident, Department of Surgery, The University of North Carolina at Chapel Hill, Chapel Hill, North Carolina

CAROLYN MENENDEZ, MD
Assistant Professor, Department of Surgery, Duke University Medical Center, Clinical Cancer Genetics, Duke Cancer Institute, Durham, North Carolina

HALEY A. MOSS, MD
Assistant Professor, Department of Obstetrics and Gynecology, Duke University Medical Center, Durham, North Carolina

BARNABAS OBENG-GYASI, BS
Senior Research Assistant, Department of Radiology, Duke University Medical Center, Durham, North Carolina

SAMILIA OBENG-GYASI, MD, MPH
Assistant Professor of Surgery, Division of Surgical Oncology, Department of Surgery, The Ohio State University, Columbus, Ohio

ALEXANDER A. PARIKH, MD, MPH
Professor and Division Chief, Division of Surgical Oncology, Department of Surgery, Brody School of Medicine at East Carolina University, Greenville, North Carolina

JENNIFER K. PLICHTA, MD, MS
Associate Professor, Departments of Surgery and Population Health Sciences, Duke University Medical Center, Durham, North Carolina

REBECCA A. SNYDER, MD, MPH
Assistant Professor, Division of Surgical Oncology, Department of Surgery, Brody School of Medicine at East Carolina University, Greenville, North Carolina

BROOKE A. STEWART
Department of Psychology, Appalachian State University, Boone, North Carolina

JOHN H. STEWART IV, MD, MBA
Professor of Surgery, Louisiana State University, New Orleans School of Medicine, Director, Louisiana State University New Orleans - Louisiana Children's Medical Center Cancer Center, New Orleans, Louisiana

WILLI TARVER, DrPH, MLIS
Assistant Professor, Division of Cancer Prevention and Control, Department of Internal Medicine, College of Medicine, The Ohio State University, Columbus, Ohio

MADELINE B. TORRES, MD
Resident, General Surgery, Department of Surgery, Penn State Health Milton S. Hershey Medical Center, Hershey, Pennsylvania

ELIZABETH WIGNALL, MS
Certified Genetic Counselor, Clinical Cancer Genetics, Duke Cancer Institute, Durham, North Carolina

Contents

> Oncologists are often ill-prepared for patient-provider communication
> about the financial costs and burden of treatment. Several barriers to
> cost communication exist, including provider discomfort, lack of knowl-
> edge or access to accurate information, and background historic concerns
> that cost discussions may negatively impact the doctor-patient relation-
> ship. However, clear and transparent cost communication can yield
> cost-reducing strategies that ultimately mitigate the high costs of cancer
> care and risk for financial toxicity.

> Over the past half century, palliative care has grown to become a pillar of
> clinical oncology. Its practice revolves around relieving suffering and opti-
> mizing quality of life, not just dealing with end-of-life decisions. Despite ev-
> idence that palliative care has the potential to reduce health care utilization
> and improve advance care planning without affecting mortality, palliative
> care remains inequitably accessible and underutilized. Furthermore, it is
> still too often introduced late in the care of patients receiving surgical inter-
> vention. This article summarizes the numerous and complex barriers to
> equitable palliative care utilization among patients with cancer. Potential
> strategies for dismantling these barriers are also discussed.

> Demographic shifts in the Unites States population highlight the growing
> need for a diverse physician workforce to care for communities of color
> and to eliminate existing disparities in cancer care and outcomes for these
> potentially vulnerable patients. The current surgical oncology workforce
> lacks adequate racial and ethnic representation, and the pool of medical
> students and surgical trainees who are underrepresented in medicine
> (URM) is scant. This review critically evaluates data, summarizes chal-
> lenges in the recruitment and retention of URM surgeons to surgical
> oncology, and provides strategies to address these workforce deficits.

Neighborhood has significant implications for breast cancer screening, stage, treatment, and mortality. Patients residing in neighborhoods with high deprivation or rurality face barriers and challenges to accessing and receiving care. Consequently, they experience higher mortality rates than their financially affluent or urban counterparts. There are multiple gaps in the literature on the relationship between place of residence and the use of systemic therapies or emerging surgical strategies for disease management. As the management of breast cancer continues to evolve, additional studies are needed to understand the implications of place on the implementation and dissemination of new and emerging treatment modalities.

Although integrated health care has largely been associated with increases in prices and static or decreased quality across many disease states, it has shown some successes in improving cancer care. However, its impact is largely equivocal, making consensus statements difficult. Critically, integration does not necessarily translate to clinical coordination, which might be the true driver behind the success of integrated health care delivery. Moving forward, it is important to establish payment models that support clinical care coordination. Shifting from a fragmented health system to a coordinated one may improve evidence-based cancer care, outcomes, and value for patients.

Genetic testing offers providers a potentially life saving tool for identifying and intervening in high-risk individuals. However, disparities in receipt of genetic testing have been consistently demonstrated and undoubtedly have significant implications for the populations not receiving the standard of care. If correctly used, there is the potential for genetic testing to play a role in decreasing health disparities among individuals of different races and ethnicities. However, if genetic testing continues to revolutionize cancer care while being disproportionately distributed, it also has the potential to widen the existing mortality gap between various racial and ethnic populations.

SURGICAL ONCOLOGY CLINICS OF NORTH AMERICA

FORTHCOMING ISSUES

April 2022
Colorectal Cancer
Traci L. Hedrick, *Editor*

July 2022
Sarcoma
Chandrajit P. Raut and Alessandro Gronchi, *Editors*

October 2022
Oncology Imaging: Updates and Advancements
Natalie Lui, *Editor*

RECENT ISSUES

October 2021
Management of Pancreatic Cancer
Susan Tsai and Douglas B. Evans, *Editors*

July 2021
Palliative Care in Surgical Oncology
Bridget N. Fahy, *Editor*

April 2021
Pediatric Cancer
Roshni Dasgupta, *Editor*

SERIES OF RELATED INTEREST

Surgical Clinics of North America
http://www.surgical.theclinics.com
Thoracic Surgery Clinics
http://www.thoracic.theclinics.com
Advances in Surgery
http://www.advancessurgery.com

THE CLINICS ARE AVAILABLE ONLINE!
Access your subscription at:
www.theclinics.com

Foreword

Disparities and Determinants of Health in Surgical Oncology

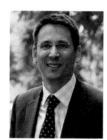

Timothy M. Pawlik, MD, MPH, MTS, PhD, FACS, FRACS (Hon.)
Consulting Editor

Traditionally, *Surgical Oncology Clinics of North America* has focused on disease- or organ-specific cancer topics. In identifying topics for this year's issues, I believed that it was critical to address disparities and determinants of health within the larger field of surgical oncology itself. As such, this issue of the *Surgical Oncology Clinics of North America* is particularly important. Like all of you, I believe we are obligated as medical professionals to address disparities, and to use our collective voice to foster awareness around disparities within oncologic care. In turn, we wanted to be purposeful in having a specific issue of *Surgical Oncology Clinics of North America* that addressed diversity, equity, and inclusion within the context of surgical oncology.

Multiple previous studies have identified race, socioeconomic status, as well as insurance status as factors that are strongly associated with cancer-specific outcomes, including receipt of guideline-compliant care, risk of perioperative morbidity and mortality, as well as differences in long-term disease-specific survival. In fact, social circumstances and environmental exposures are among the most important contributors to early death in the United States. Social determinants of health have been defined by the World Health Organization as the conditions in which people are born, grow, live, work, and age. These determinants can include factors such as housing, transportation, education, employment, and access to care. The COVID-19 pandemic only served to lay bare even more how race/ethnicity, privilege, and social determinants of health all so often dictate health care outcomes and access to care. In light of this, I am grateful to have Dr Oluwadamilola M. Fayanju as the guest editor of this important issue of *Surgical Oncology Clinics of North America*. Dr Fayanju is the Helen O. Dickens Presidential Associate Professor and Chief of Breast Surgery at Penn Medicine, University of Pennsylvania Health System. Dr Fayanju obtained her medical degree at Washington University in St. Louis, where she also subsequently completed her residency. Dr Fayanju then completed a Breast Fellowship at the University of

Surg Oncol Clin N Am 31 (2022) xi–xii
https://doi.org/10.1016/j.soc.2021.09.001
1055-3207/22/© 2021 Published by Elsevier Inc.

Texas MD Anderson Cancer Center. Dr Fayanju has a strong and long-standing commitment to promoting equity and efficacy with which breast cancer patients are treated, a guiding principle that is reflected in her clinical practice and research endeavors. She is an academic breast surgeon who conducts health services research focused on addressing disparities in breast cancer outcome and treatment as well as improving the quality and efficiency of breast cancer care delivery using the principles of value-based health care. As such, Dr Fayanju is imminently qualified to be the guest editor of this important issue of *Surgical Oncology Clinics of North America.*

The issue covers a number of important topics, including financial toxicity, barriers to equitable palliative care, as well as how bias and disparities impact access to care for pancreatic, breast, colorectal and, among others, peritoneal cancers. In addition, the issue also tackles other important topics, such as disparities in recruiting and retaining a diverse surgical oncology team, as well as the challenge of implementing integrated health care systems into oncology care to improve outcomes for all. Furthermore, the topic of disparities in clinical trials, as well as proposals and solutions to tackle this challenge, is presented. In sum, the talented group of authors amassed by Dr Fayanju holistically addresses issues of diversity and disparity related to patient care, as well as the health care team and the health care delivery system.

I am very grateful to Dr Fayanju for her work in identifying such a wonderful group of oncology leaders to contribute to this issue of *Surgical Oncology Clinics of North America.* The team of authors has done a skillful job of highlighting the importance of diversity, as well as the need to incorporate attention to social determinants of health into the care of all our cancer patients. I am convinced that this issue of *Surgical Oncology Clinics of North America* will serve us well to help identify ways in which we can address disparities in cancer care that, it is hoped, will lead to addressing and eliminating persistent inequities. I would like to thank Dr Fayanju and all the contributing authors again for an important issue of the *Surgical Oncology Clinics of North America* that should inform how we care for all our patients with cancer.

Timothy M. Pawlik, MD, MPH, MTS, PhD, FACS, FRACS (Hon.)
Department of Surgery
The Urban Meyer III and Shelley Meyer Chair for Cancer Research
Departments of Surgery, Oncology, and Health Services Management and Policy
The Ohio State University Wexner Medical Center
395 West 12th Avenue, Suite 670
Columbus, OH 43210, USA

E-mail address:
tim.pawlik@osumc.edu

Preface

Surgical Oncology for All: Why We Must Prioritize Inclusion and Equity for Our Patients and Ourselves

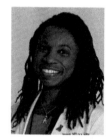

Oluwadamilola M. Fayanju, MD, MA, MPHS, FACS
Editor

Cancer does not happen in a vacuum. Behind every patient with cancer is a story, and attached to every cancer diagnosis are real people, humans changed by the unwelcome discovery of the Big C in their own body or that of a loved one. But at the dawn of 2020, the C word at the center of our professional world was supplanted by another, buoyed aloft on a wave of fear and uncertainty. This new entity, COVID-19, has redefined our lexicon and our planet, and on arrival, it completely upended the provision of oncologic care around the world.

We stopped performing "elective" cases. We halted screening. We pivoted to less conventional care pathways, as we sought to find a way forward for those unlucky enough to be diagnosed with cancer in the midst of a global pandemic. We became intensivists and phlebotomists, organizers of home school and virtual conferences. We made mistakes, and we made amends. We prayed for vaccines, and we wept with relief when we received them.

And we mourned. We mourned the millions of lives worldwide that COVID-19 has taken from us. We mourned the unrealized unity that has eluded our country, as mask-wearing and other public health measures were mocked, politicized, and ignored by those who should know better. And we mourned the many patients with cancer that we never met, the individuals for whom job loss and childcare and bankruptcy caused screenings to be skipped and symptoms to be ignored.

The outsized effect the pandemic has had on communities of color laid bare the long-standing inequities in housing, income, employment, and other social determinants of health that fueled observed disparities in COVID-19-related morbidity and

Surg Oncol Clin N Am 31 (2022) xiii–xiv
https://doi.org/10.1016/j.soc.2021.08.005
1055-3207/22/© 2021 Published by Elsevier Inc.

mortality. It gave voice to the long-simmering rage felt in so many black and brown communities, as a new viral scourge raged through homes and neighborhoods already strained to the point of breaking. The pandemic also shed light on the vitriol that has long been endured by members of the Asian community in this country and that has, unfortunately, flourished as those inclined to imbibe hateful misinformation suddenly felt emboldened to act upon it. Finally, the importance of recruiting, retaining, and supporting physicians of color and an acknowledgement of the role that systemic racism has played in perpetuating their underrepresentation in medicine were universally embraced by professional societies within and beyond surgery, groups who also, often for the first time, took concrete steps toward eliminating these gaps in equity.

In response to our changed and changing world, I have had the great honor of serving as the guest editor for the latest issue of *Surgical Oncology Clinics of North America*, titled "Disparities and Determinants of Health in Surgical Oncology." In this issue, our colleagues review a number of topics reflected in this issue's title, ranging from disparities in receipt of palliative care and participation in clinical trials to disease-specific examples of disparate treatment and outcome. We also examine the structural features of our healthcare system (e.g., fragmentation and suboptimal integration of care) that contribute to financial toxicity and treatment non-adherence. Most importantly, we offer concrete steps for change.

Our great talent as surgeons is the ability to innovate and adapt in response to new data, unfamiliar terrain, and unexpected circumstances. Now, as we face the most significant public health crisis of our generation, we have an obligation to make the most of this talent and to channel this crisis into building a more just world for our patients, our neighbors, and ourselves.

Oluwadamilola M. Fayanju, MD, MA, MPHS, FACS
Department of Surgery
Rena Rowan Breast Center
Abramson Cancer Center
Perelman School of Medicine at the
University of Pennsylvania/Penn Medicine
3400 Spruce Street
Silverstein 4
Philadelphia, PA 19104, USA

E-mail address:
Oluwadamilola.Fayanju@pennmedicine.upenn.edu

Twitter: @DrLolaFayanju (O.M. Fayanju)

Financial Toxicity and Shared Decision Making in Oncology

Rachel A. Greenup, MD, MPH[a,b,*]

KEYWORDS

- Cancer • Disparities • Financial toxicity • Shared decision making

KEY POINTS

- Financial toxicity is now recognized as a major side effect of cancer care and is experienced by up to 70% of patients and their families.
- Cancer-related financial hardship has been associated with poor physical and mental well-being, treatment nonadherence, a greater risk of bankruptcy, and early death.
- For patients with cancer, the initial surgical consultation is often when individuals and their families begin learning about their treatment options and making choices regarding their oncology care. However, we as surgical oncologists are often ill-prepared for patient-provider communication about the financial costs and burden of treatment.
- Cost transparency and communication in shared cancer decisions may protect patients against financial hardship and yield cost-reducing strategies, including coordination of appointments, purchasing supplemental insurance, and applying for charity care to cover high deductibles, which ultimately mitigate the high costs of cancer care and risk for financial toxicity.

FINANCIAL TOXICITY AMONG PATIENTS WITH CANCER

Rising health care costs have resulted in significant financial hardship for individuals with cancer. From 2010 to 2020, health care expenditures in the United States related to cancer care increased by 27% and were projected to reach $180 billion based on population growth alone.[1] Large health system expenditures have translated into cost sharing, resulting in more frequent and more costly deductibles and copayments for individuals undergoing treatment.[1–5] As a result, financial hardship is now recognized as a major side effect of cancer care and is experienced by up to 70% of patients and their families.[6,7] Cancer-related financial hardship has been associated with poor

[a] Division of Surgical Oncology, Department of Surgery, Yale University School of Medicine, 310 Cedar Street, LH 118, New Haven, CT 60510, USA; [b] The Breast Center at Smilow Cancer Hospital at Yale New Haven, New Haven, CT 06511, USA
* Division of Surgical Oncology, Department of Surgery, Yale University School of Medicine, 310 Cedar Street, LH 118, New Haven, CT 60510.
E-mail address: rachel.greenup@yale.edu

Surg Oncol Clin N Am 31 (2022) 1–7
https://doi.org/10.1016/j.soc.2021.08.001
1055-3207/22/© 2021 Elsevier Inc. All rights reserved.

physical and mental well-being, treatment nonadherence, a greater risk of bankruptcy, and early death.[7–10] Cancer-related financial hardship impacts patient quality of life, receipt of life-saving therapies, and survival.

The substantial economic burden of national cancer care varies by cancer type, geographic region, and extent of health care utilization. From 1998 to 2000, mean monthly cancer-related expenditures ranged from $2187 for prostate cancer to $7616 for pancreatic cancer compared with monthly medical expenses of $329 for matched controls without cancer.[11] For patients and caregivers, the burden of cancer-related financial costs includes direct payments for medical care, indirect costs related to lost productivity and employment disruption, and the hidden costs of travel, lodging, and time that remain poorly characterized.[7,8,11–14] A 2016 systematic review published by Altice and colleagues[15] evaluated articles (N = 676) published between 1990 and 2015 that described the financial experiences of cancer survivors. In this study, financial hardship was reported as material conditions (eg, out-of-pocket payments, productivity loss, medical debt, or bankruptcy), psychological responses (eg, distress or worry), and coping behaviors. Overall, mean annual productivity loss ranged from $380 to $8236, 12% to 62% of cancer survivors reported debt related to cancer treatment, 47% to 49% reported experiencing financial distress, and 4% to 45% reported nonadherence to cancer medication due to cost.[15]

Notably, the average out-of-pocket payments for cancer treatment are higher than costs for other noncancer medical diagnoses and can be unaffordable even in the insured. Risk factors for financial hardship include young age, being ineligible for Medicare, non-Hispanic black race, low income, and unpartnered or single marital status.[6,11,13,14,16,17] Prior research has demonstrated that 25% to almost half (46%) of insured patients with cancer spend much of their savings to pay for treatment and many reduce spending on basic needs to afford their cancer care.[7] Among insured adults taking oral anticancer therapy, unexpected financial burden (odds ratio [OR], 2.89; 95% confidence interval [CI], 1.41 to 5.89; $P<.01$) and distress (OR, 1.64; 95% CI, 1.38–1.96; $P<.01$) were associated with an increased the risk of medication nonadherence.[18] Although the overwhelming majority of patients with cancer meet their deductibles shortly after diagnosis, cumulative premiums, deductibles, and out-of-pocket maximums (ranging from $1000–$10,000) that reset each calendar year can be unrelenting.

Notably, racial and ethnic minorities are disproportionately at risk of cancer-related financial hardship. In a survey from the Carolina Breast Cancer Program, Wheeler and colleagues[19] demonstrated that black women reported a significantly greater financial impact of their cancer diagnosis when compared with whites (58% vs 40%, $P<.001$) across several domains, including (1) decrease in income (49% vs 35%, $P<.001$), (2) financial barrier to care (24% vs 11%, $P<.001$), (3) transportation barrier to care (14% vs 3%, $P<.001$), (4) lost job as a result of cancer (14% vs 3%, $P<.001$), and (5) loss of health insurance (5% vs 1%, $P<.001$). Notably, the existing literature also demonstrates that strategies to cope with cancer-related financial hardship also differ based on patient race and ethnicity; non-Hispanic black individuals are more likely to stop or refuse treatment as coping strategies to mitigate financial hardship when compared with whites.[20]

Moreover, individuals with cancer are at an increased risk of short-term disability and a 4-fold greater risk of work absenteeism when compared with matched controls.[11] In a nationally represented survey of women (N = 1628) enrolled in the Sister Study or Two Sisters Study, 27% of participants employed at diagnosis experienced employment disruption (15% stopped work completely; 12% reported working fewer hours after diagnosis) and 21% reported experiencing financial hardship (16% had difficulty paying for care; 12.6% borrowed money or incurred debt).[21] Not surprisingly, employment disruption was associated with an almost 2-fold risk of financial hardship.

The continuum of cancer care is a lengthy and demanding process. The initial phase of cancer treatment typically consists of costly diagnostic evaluations followed by treatment, such as chemotherapy, hormonal therapy, surgery, and radiation. More recently, effective yet expensive targeted therapies have been added to adjuvant regimens, further contributing to financial strain.[22–24] Receipt of care across several sub-specialty teams can exacerbate the complex logistical challenges required to access multidisciplinary cancer treatment[25]; this is especially true for the most vulnerable patients with cancer, including children and those with the rarest tumor types; when care cannot be provided closer to home, expenses associated with relocation to obtain treatment at medical centers capable of providing complex cancer care translates into an even greater financial sacrifice.[13,15,22,26,27]

The growing population of individuals living with metastatic cancer remains highly vulnerable to cancer-related financial hardship. In a small survey of women with metastatic breast cancer (N = 84), Williams and colleagues[21] established that although low health literacy was not independently associated with financial hardship, it correlated with greater material and behavioral financial hardship. Participants with low health literacy more often reported borrowing money (19% vs 4%), an inability to pay for food or rent (10% vs 4%), and skipping a procedure (8% vs 1%), medical test (7% vs 0%), or treatment (4% vs 0%).

For patients with cancer who undergo treatment with curative intent, surveillance and maintenance therapy can last for years and often require close monitoring and intensive health care utilization. In the United States, the growing population of cancer survivors and increased overall life expectancy has resulted in medically complex individuals living longer after oncology treatment. As a result, primary care physicians and oncologists will need to manage the side effects of cancer treatment in an aging cohort with baseline comorbid conditions, and thus, the continued survivorship phase will become increasingly costly.[28] In breast cancer survivors alone, growing health care costs among Medicare beneficiaries are expected to increase by $1 billion in the next decade.

Last, the final phase of cancer care (ie, the last 12 months of life) has historically been the costliest, with multiple studies demonstrating that these patients are disproportionately at risk of financial hardship.

COST TRANSPARENCY, PATIENT-PROVIDER COMMUNICATION, AND SHARED DECISION MAKING IN ONCOLOGY

In 2009, the American Society of Clinical Oncology encouraged oncologists to discuss the costs of care with individuals embarking on treatment.[29] More recently, the Institute of Medicine proposed that patient-provider cost communication and personal spending burden be considered as national metrics for high-quality health care.[30,31] Despite these high-level endorsements, existing literature has suggested that cost transparency and communication are rarely included in shared cancer treatment decisions.[32,33] The extent to which cancer diagnosis and treatment impacts financial security depends on financial well-being at the time of diagnosis, including insurance coverage, savings, and job security; however, efforts are being made to improve cost transparency and communication as part of shared decision making.

The combined literature demonstrates that more than 75% of prompted oncologists believe that patients should have access to cost information, yet only 30% include cost discussions as part of their routine clinical practice.[32–34] In an era of financial toxicity, cost transparency and communication remain lacking in clinical cancer treatment decisions. On cross-sectional survey of insured patients with cancer (N = 300) receiving treatment, more than one-third (39%) reported higher-than-expected financial burden from cancer care and 16% reported high or overwhelming financial distress.[13] Multiple validated decision tools have been studied in this setting, and their use has been associated with improved decision quality and satisfaction.[35–37] Yet, the financial costs and care burden remain largely absent from decision science and clinical care. In 2009, the American Society of Clinical Oncology endorsed patient-provider cost communication as a potential solution[29]; yet a decade later, cost discussions remain rare in clinical oncology and effective interventions targeting financial toxicity remain lacking.

The initial surgical consultation is often a patient's first point of contact with their cancer team, where affected individuals and their families begin learning about their treatment options and making choices regarding their oncology care. Thus, surgeons' knowledge of and awareness around the impact of financial toxicity is important when caring for oncology patients. Financial insecurity in patients with cancer has been associated with downstream nonadherence and refusal of treatment[38]; early treatment decisions that result in high patient costs have the potential to influence the receipt of subsequent treatment. Cost transparency and communication in shared cancer decisions may protect patients against financial hardship along the entire continuum of oncology care and improve long-term adherence to recommended multimodal therapy.[39]

Growing evidence suggests that value is added in the oncology setting with improved efforts around cost transparency and communication.[7,33,34,40,41] In a national survey of US oncologists, surgical oncologists reported that common barriers to cost discussions included inaccessible cost information, lack of knowledge, and a perceived inability to intervene.[33] Importantly, 36% of providers believed that patients with cancer would have a negative view of cost discussions; however, early research has demonstrated that cost communication is feasible, acceptable, and desired by patients with cancer.[7,42,43] In outpatient breast oncology appointments, 50% of cost conversations resulted in cost-reducing strategies.[42] Physicians offered less expensive treatment options, altered timing of interventions to coincide with insurance coverage, and connected patients to local philanthropic resources for financial support.[42] Patients similarly used cost-reducing strategies such as coordinating appointments, purchasing supplemental insurance, and applying for charity care.

Following completion of treatment, the overwhelming majority of cancer survivors wished they had access to cost information when making cancer treatment decisions. However, cost information and the potential for financial toxicity may be difficult to process at the time of a cancer diagnosis; the distress of a life-threatening diagnosis takes priority over monetary strategy, navigating insurance, and protection of employment.[16] Young age, minority race, lower household income (<$70,000/y), receipt of multimodal therapy, and advanced stage at diagnosis are associated with an increased risk of financial toxicity.[10,11,22] Notably, wealth and adequate insurance coverage are not entirely protective. Regardless of socioeconomic status before diagnosis, all patients with cancer and their families are vulnerable to the devastating financial burden of cancer diagnosis and treatment.[12]

FUTURE DIRECTIONS

Oncologists are ill-prepared for patient-provider communication about the financial costs and burden of treatment. Several barriers to cost communication exist, including provider discomfort, lack of knowledge or access to accurate information, and background historic concerns that cost discussions may negatively impact the doctor-patient relationship.[13] However, existing literature has suggested that cost communication has resulted in cost-reducing strategies that ultimately mitigate the high costs of cancer care; these include coordination of appointments, purchasing supplemental insurance, and applying for charity care to cover high deductibles.[7,42,43] Communication about financial costs and health care burden has the potential to be challenging in clinical cancer care, because cost transparency and communication may be distressing for patients at the time of a life-threatening diagnosis. It is important, however, to make resources available at the institutional and health system levels to support oncology patients' psychosocial and financial needs during treatment and beyond.

Although a given patient's cost awareness is not independently sufficient to solve the crisis of financial toxicity, increased and early cost transparency may activate patients to improve understanding and expectations, motivate cost communication and preparedness, and empower advocacy around cancer-related financial hardship. Including cost information as part of shared cancer treatment decisions promises to (1) provide information, (2) connect individuals to resources, (3) promote peer discussions within and across communities, and (4) change social norms.[44,45] Improved communication regarding the risk of financial toxicity in shared oncology treatment decisions has the potential to improve the quality of these decisions and to prepare patients for the financial costs and nonmonetary burden of cancer treatment.

Altered communication regarding this growing and meaningful side effect of oncology treatment posits to enhance shared cancer treatment decisions, reduce the risk of financial hardship, and improve patient-centered care.

DISCLOSURE

Nothing to disclose.

REFERENCES

1. Mariotto AB, Yabroff KR, Shao Y, et al. Projections of the cost of cancer care in the United States: 2010-2020. J Natl Cancer Inst 2011;103(2):117–28.
2. Yabroff KR, Lund J, Kepka D, et al. Economic burden of cancer in the United States: estimates, projections, and future research. Cancer Epidemiol Biomarkers Prev 2011;20(10):2006–14.
3. Lorenzoni L, Belloni A, Sassi F. Health-care expenditure and health policy in the USA versus other high-spending OECD countries. Lancet 2014;384(9937):83–92.
4. Elkin EB, Bach PB. Cancer's next frontier: addressing high and increasing costs. JAMA 2010;303(11):1086–7.
5. Himmelstein DU, Woolhandler S, Almberg M, et al. The U.S. health care crisis continues: a data snapshot. Int J Health Serv 2018;48(1):28–41.
6. Zafar Y, Abernethy AP, Tulsky JA, et al. Financial distress, communication, and cancer treatment decision making: does cost matter? J Clin Oncol 2013; 31(15_suppl):6506.
7. Zafar SY, Abernethy AP. Financial toxicity, Part I: a new name for a growing problem. Oncology (Williston Park) 2013;27(2):80–1, 149.
8. Tucker-Seeley RD, Yabroff KR. Minimizing the "Financial Toxicity" associated with cancer care: advancing the research agenda. J Natl Cancer Inst 2016;108(5): djv410.

9. Ramsey SD, Bansal A, Fedorenko CR, et al. Financial insolvency as a risk factor for early mortality among patients with cancer. J Clin Oncol 2016;34(9):980–6.

10. Kale HP, Carroll NV. Self-reported financial burden of cancer care and its effect on physical and mental health-related quality of life among US cancer survivors. Cancer 2016;122(8):283–9.

11. Chang S, Long SR, Kutikova L, et al. Estimating the cost of cancer: results on the basis of claims data analyses for cancer patients diagnosed with seven types of cancer during 1999 to 2000. J Clin Oncol 2004;22(17):3524.

12. Rice DP. Estimating the cost of illness. Am J Public Health Nations Health 1967; 57(3):424–40.

13. Chino F, Peppercorn JM, Rushing C, et al. Out-of-pocket costs, financial distress, and underinsurance in cancer care. JAMA Oncol 2017;3(11):1582–4.

14. Banegas MP, Guy GP Jr, de Moor JS, et al. For working-age cancer survivors, medical debt and bankruptcy create financial hardships. Health Aff (Millwood) 2016;35(1):54–61.

15. Altice CK, Banegas MP, Tucker-Seeley RD, et al. Financial hardships experienced by cancer survivors: a systematic review. J Natl Cancer Inst 2017;109(2):djw205.

16. Greenup RA, Fish L, Campbell BM, et al. Financial costs and burden related to decisions for breast cancer surgery. J Oncol Pract 2019;15(8):e666–76.

17. Bernard DSM, Farr SL, Fang Z. National estimates of out-of-pocket health care expenditure burdens among nonelderly adults with cancer: 2001 to 2008. J Clin Oncol 2011;29(20):2821–6.

18. Bestvina CM, Zullig LL, Rushing C, et al. Patient-oncologist cost communication, financial distress, and medication adherence. J Oncol Pract 2014;10(3):162–7.

19. Wheeler SB, Spencer JC, Pinheiro LC, et al. Financial impact of breast cancer in black versus white women. J Clin Oncol 2018;36(17):1695–701.

20. Samuel CA, Spencer JC, Rosenstein DL, et al. Racial differences in employment and cost-management behaviors in patients with metastatic breast cancer. Breast Cancer Res Treat 2020;179(1):207–15.

21. Meernik C, Sandler DP, Peipins LA, et al. Breast cancer–related employment disruption and financial hardship in the sister study. JNCI Cancer Spectr 2021; 5(3):pkab024.

22. Green DM, Breslow NE, Beckwith JB, et al. Effect of duration of treatment on treatment outcome and cost of treatment for Wilms' tumor: a report from the National Wilms' Tumor Study Group. J Clin Oncol 1998;16(12):3744–51.

23. Kalapurakal JA, Dome JS, Perlman EJ, et al. Management of Wilms' tumour: current practice and future goals. Lancet Oncol 2004;5(1):37–46.

24. Varan A. Wilms' tumor in children: an overview. Nephron Clin Pract 2008;108(2): c83–90.

25. Bona K, Dussel V, Orellana L, et al. Economic impact of advanced pediatric cancer on families. J Pain Symptom Manage 2014;47(3):594–603.

26. Albritton KH, Wiggins CH, Nelson HE, et al. Site of oncologic specialty care for older adolescents in Utah. J Clin Oncol 2007;25(29):4616–21.

27. Santacroce SJ, Kneipp SM. A conceptual model of financial toxicity in pediatric oncology. J Pediatr Oncol Nurs 2019;36(1):6–16.

28. Yashkin AP, Greenup RA, Gorbunova G, et al. Outcomes and costs for women after breast cancer: preparing for improved survivorship of medicare beneficiaries. JCO Oncol Pract 2020;17(4):e469–78.

29. Meropol NJ, Schrag D, Smith TJ, et al. American Society of clinical oncology guidance statement: the cost of cancer care. J Clin Oncol 2009;27(23):3868–74.

30. Blumenthal D, McGinnis JM. Measuring vital signs: an IOM report on core metrics for health and health care progress. JAMA 2015;313(19):1901–2.
31. Committee on improving the quality of cancer care: addressing the challenges of an aging P, Board on Health Care S, Institute of M. In: Levit L, Balogh E, Nass S, et al, editors. Delivering high-quality cancer care: charting a new course for a system in crisis. National Academies Press (US) Copyright 2013 by the National Academy of Sciences. All rights reserved; 2013.
32. Greenup RA, Rushing CR, Peppercorn J, et al. Perspectives on the costs of cancer care: a survey of the American Society of Breast Surgeons. Ann Surg Oncol 2019;26(10):3141–51.
33. Altomare I, Irwin B, Zafar SY, et al. ReCAP: physician experience and attitudes toward addressing the cost of cancer care. J Oncol Pract 2016;12(3):247–8.
34. Shih YT, Chien CR. A review of cost communication in oncology: Patient attitude, provider acceptance, and outcome assessment. Cancer 2017;123(6):928–39.
35. Sepucha K, Ozanne E, Silvia K, et al. An approach to measuring the quality of breast cancer decisions. Patient Educ Couns 2007;65(2):261–9.
36. Lee CN, Chang Y, Adimorah N, et al. Decision making about surgery for early-stage breast cancer. J Am Coll Surg 2012;214(1):1–10.
37. Whelan T, Levine M, Willan A, et al. Effect of a decision aid on knowledge and treatment decision making for breast cancer surgery: a randomized trial. JAMA 2004;292(4):435–41.
38. Hastert TA, Banegas MP, Hamel LM, et al. Race, financial hardship, and limiting care due to cost in a diverse cohort of cancer survivors. J Cancer Surviv 2019; 13(3):429–37.
39. Wan C, Williams CP, Nipp RD, et al. Treatment decision making and financial toxicity in women with metastatic breast cancer. Clin Breast Cancer 2021;21(1): 37–46.
40. Bullock AJ, Hofstatter EW, Yushak ML, et al. Understanding patients' attitudes toward communication about the cost of cancer care. J Oncol Pract 2012;8(4): e50–8.
41. Greenup RA, Rushing CN, Fish LJ, et al. Perspectives on the costs of cancer care: a survey of the American Society of breast surgeons. Ann Surg Oncol 2019;26(10):3141–51.
42. Hunter WG, Zafar SY, Hesson A, et al. Discussing health care expenses in the oncology clinic: analysis of cost conversations in outpatient encounters. J Oncol Pract 2017;13(11):e944–56.
43. Greenup RA, Rushing CR, Peppercorn J, et al. The costs of breast cancer care: patient-reported experiences and preferences for transparency 2017.
44. Wilkin HA, Ball-Rokeach SJ. Reaching at risk groups: the importance of health storytelling in Los Angeles Latino media. Journalism 2006;7(3):299–320.
45. Patient voices programme. Available at: www.patientvoices.org.uk.

Barriers to Equitable Palliative Care Utilization Among Patients with Cancer

Gabriel D. Ivey, MD[a], Fabian M. Johnston, MD, MHS[b],*

KEYWORDS

- Barriers to palliative care • Cancer • Hospice and palliative medicine
- Palliative care disparities

KEY POINTS

- The mission of palliative care is to relieve suffering and optimize quality of life, not just deal with end-of-life decisions.
- Palliative care is inequitably accessible, underutilized, and often introduced late in the care of patients receiving surgical intervention.
- Existing barriers to equitable palliative care utilization among patients with cancer are numerous and complex.
- Dismantling current barriers to equitable palliative care utilization among patients with cancer will require coordinated efforts at the level of both providers and professional organizations.

INTRODUCTION

Palliative care (PC) has become a pillar of clinical oncology. As a community of surgeons who have dedicated careers to fighting cancer and alleviating suffering, we must acknowledge this. Patients with cancer not only deserve access to surgical, medical, and radiation oncologists when clinically appropriate but they should also be afforded PC interventions concomitantly with standard oncologic treatment. This is the current recommendation of the American Society of Clinical Oncology (ASCO).[1] It is the product of significant progress in the development and growth of PC services over the past half century.[2] Medicine is increasingly realizing the true mission of PC—to relieve suffering and optimize quality of life, not just deal with end-of-life decisions. The practice of PC affirms life and regards death as normal,

[a] Department of Surgery, Division of Surgical Oncology, The Johns Hopkins University, 600 North Wolfe Street, Blalock 611, Baltimore, MD 21287, USA; [b] Department of Surgery, Division of Surgical Oncology, The Johns Hopkins University, 600 North Wolfe Street, Blalock 606, Baltimore, MD 21287, USA
* Corresponding author.
E-mail address: fjohnst4@jhmi.edu

Surg Oncol Clin N Am 31 (2022) 9–20
https://doi.org/10.1016/j.soc.2021.07.003
1055-3207/22/© 2021 Elsevier Inc. All rights reserved.

and in this context, practitioners seek neither to hasten nor to postpone the dying process.[3]

Unfortunately, PC remains inequitably accessible, underutilized, and is still too often introduced late in the care of patients receiving surgical intervention,[4] despite evidence that PC has the potential to reduce health care utilization and improve advance care planning (ACP) without affecting mortality.[5] People of color are particularly at risk for suboptimal access to and utilization of PC,[6] a byproduct of America's history of systemic racism, which has long served as a barrier to equitable health care.[7] Additional barriers are numerous and complex. They include lack of PC training for most clinicians,[8] inadequate knowledge regarding indications and data on triggers for PC referrals,[9] a paucity of PC specialists,[10] and poor communication between physicians and patients.[11,12] Foundational to these barriers is the misconception held by both patients and clinicians that PC is equivalent to terminal care.[13]

In this article the authors discuss current barriers to equitable PC utilization for patients with cancer and provide recommendations for how these barriers can be dismantled.

BARRIERS TO EQUITABLE PALLIATIVE CARE UTILIZATION

Barriers to equitable PC utilization among patients with cancer are numerous and complex. With racism having long served as a barrier to equitable health care, correlations between patient race and likelihood of PC underutilization have been observed, especially African Americans.[7] Other marginalized populations—including sexual and gender minorities, people with disabilities, children, and the elderly—have also faced structural, social, and economic barriers, which have in turn also impaired utilization of PC interventions when clinically appropriate.[14–17] The evidence for disparity within most of these populations, however, is scarce and as such, the following discussion focuses primarily on the data surrounding African Americans.

Additional barriers are in large part the result of our health care system's failure to reconcile with the pillar of clinical oncology that PC has become and can be subsumed under 1 of 3 categories: (1) gaps in knowledge, (2) training deficits, and (3) poor communication among providers and between providers and patients. These barriers are further detailed in the sections that follow.

RACE AND RACISM IN PALLIATIVE CARE ACCESS AND PROVISION

Racism has long served as a barrier to equitable health care, and, as previously acknowledged by the Society of Surgical Oncology (SSO), it underpins many of the health disparities observed in our field.[7,18] Unsurprisingly, it is also a determinant of PC utilization,[6,19–27] particularly for African American patients with cancer. Studies show that African Americans are less likely to participate in ACP,[20] enroll in hospice care,[21,22] and have discussions regarding prognosis.[25] They are also more likely to have a higher symptom burden,[19] not understand their illness or treatment goals,[28] and pursue life-sustaining therapies regardless of prognosis.[29]

Advance care planning[20,30–32]—a communication process through which people plan for when they cannot make their own medical decisions in the form of a living will, durable power of attorney for health care decision-making (health care proxy), and/or Do-Not-Resuscitate (DNR) documentation—is often considered a correlate for PC utilization, as it provides a template for patients to discuss end-of-life care with their loved ones and physicians.[33] It is unclear why African Americans have substantially lower rates of ACP despite current national guidelines recommending ACP, including discussions about PC and hospice.[34] A study by Smith and colleagues examined whether sociocultural differences, such as acknowledgment of terminal illness and religiousness, explained observed disparities.[31] They found no association with current observations.

Other attributed causes for racial and ethnic differences in ACP and PC utilization are wide-ranging. Numerous studies have observed that among African Americans there is a greater preference for more aggressive/high-intensity care at the end of life.[22,35] Such differences in care preferences, however, have not been found to account for inequities in PC utilization.[30,31] Others have attributed differences in PC utilization to lack of trust between racial/ethnic minorities and their providers,[36,37] but evidence for this is also lacking.[30,38] These examples highlight the challenges in this area of study. The complex interplay of historical and social experiences,[39] culture,[40] religion/spirituality,[41,42] and knowledge gaps that shape patients' views and preferences about PC have proved difficult to decode and thus require further study.

Further compounding the difficulty in identifying factors affecting PC utilization along racial lines is the fact that access to PC does not necessarily confer equitable utilization of PC interventions. Ingersoll and colleagues observed prognosis communication with PC specialists was less than half as likely to occur during conversations with Black or Latino patients compared with others.[25] Gramling and colleagues observed PC clinicians were more likely to overestimate survival for patients who identified as Black or Latino, which led to decreased hospice use.[26] Similarly, patient preferences for end-of-life care are not always followed.[27] In a cohort of 302 patients with stage IV cancer, Loggers and colleagues observed that white patients with a preference for intensive end-of-life care were 3 times more likely to receive it and have their DNR orders/end-of-life preferences followed in comparison to black patients.[27]

Research and advocacy in this arena, including the faith-based initiative EQUAL ACP,[43] are ongoing, and it is hoped that they will shed light on actionable factors that account for racial differences in PC utilization. Current disparities are undoubtedly the result of our country's history with race.[7] In the interim, while these factors are fleshed out, attention should simultaneously be paid to other systemic barriers affecting equitable PC utilization that, if dismantled, would likely also improve disparities in PC utilization among African Americans and other marginalized populations.

GAPS IN KNOWLEDGE ABOUT PALLIATIVE CARE

Despite having become a pillar of oncology, there is a dearth of knowledge with regard to PC and misunderstanding about its use—both at the provider and patient levels. For surgeons, little is known about the scope and nature of PC.[44] In addition, it is also unclear when PC should be introduced into clinical care.[44] This ignorance, which surgeons have previously acknowledged,[45] has allowed the stigma associated with PC to persist and thrive.[13,46] Providers along with patients and their families often view the utilization of PC as synonymous with being terminally ill with weeks to live.[46,47] Such gaps in PC knowledge contribute to inequitable utilization of PC services, which in turn are often associated with disparities in health outcomes.[48] It is well documented that members of ethnic and racial minority groups are disproportionately less informed about PC.[49,50] Thus, the interaction of providers and patient knowledge gaps translate into a perpetuation of existing disparities.[51]

Surgeons are not alone; PC is underutilized across all specialties.[52] Patients treated by surgeons, however, seem the most afflicted.[53,54] Surgeons are less likely to administer PC or consult PC specialists when appropriate.[53,55] Patients on surgical services are more likely to be recommended major operative intervention when there are alternatives.[55] The PC consultations surgeons typically place are more often for assistance with end-of-life discussions than for assistance with symptom management.[54,56] Many surgeons have expressed concern that if they consult PC specialists, patients and their families will think they are "giving up."[57] In turn, and contrary to current guidelines, only 20% of current specialized PC physicians receive early referrals (ie, for patients estimated to have >6-month prognosis of survival).[58]

Given this context of clear gaps in PC knowledge at the provider level, it should come as no surprise that most Americans do not know what PC is.[59] Misconceptions of it abound, even among those who report having adequate knowledge of PC.[59] Dispelling these misperceptions is undoubtedly the job of informed providers, which should in turn improve current inequities in PC utilization as most adults still consider health care providers to be their primary source for knowledge about PC.[59]

TRAINING DEFICITS AMONG PROVIDERS ABOUT PALLIATIVE CARE

The aforementioned gaps in PC knowledge are the result of an undertrained workforce. Inequitable access to and underutilization of PC are byproducts of that dynamic. Surgeons, and in particular surgical oncologists, occupy a prime position to serve as champions for PC given the care they provide to patients with life-limiting illnesses. Accordingly, the current training paradigm for surgical oncologists needs to be reexamined and reformed.

Surveys of recent Complex General Surgical Oncology (CGSO) fellowship graduates have only made more clear the magnitude of change that is needed. Only 18.6% of recent graduates report knowing how to tell a patient he or she is dying.[60] Twenty-seven percent report knowing how to discuss stopping antineoplastic therapy with a patient and changing the focus to PC.[60] Thirty-two percent report knowing how to determine when to refer patients to hospice.[60] Exposure to PC during training is critical, and at present, nearly all (98%) CGSO fellows do not have a PC rotation during fellowship. Only 50% of recent graduates reported having PC exposure during training.[60]

This lack of training is not a new phenomenon. Most surgeons in clinical practice have not received formal PC training.[11,45,61] Of the approximately 8200 physicians with formal hospice and palliative medicine (HPM) training, only 80 are surgeons,[62] demonstrating how little surgeons have been encouraged to acquire competence in PC. At present, only 2 of what might be considered the 5 preeminent surgical textbooks have at least 1 chapter dedicated to PC (Current Surgical Therapy, 13th Ed.; Schwartz's Principles of Surgery, 11th Ed. include sections on PC but Sabiston Textbook of Surgery, 20th Ed.; Greenfield's Surgery, 6th Ed.; and Fischer's Mastery of Surgery, 7th Ed. do not).[63–67] There is also no PC chapter in the current major surgical oncology textbook (Textbook of Complex General Surgical Oncology, 1st Ed).[68]

The absence of PC training model for all oncologists[67,69,70] may also be, in part, the result of there being an HPM specialty—a critically needed discipline given our aging and more chronically ill population.[71] The growing demand for PC providers, however, continues to outstrip supply.[10,72] In this context, there has been an increased push for surgical oncologists and other non-HPM specialists to obtain basic PC skillsets and embrace particular PC tenets, such as basic symptom management to help meet evolving PC needs and aligning treatments and interventions with a patient's short- and long-term goals.[73] Although these physicians—dubbed "PC Champions" by some[74]—would fill in the gaps for more basic PC needs, complex PC tasks, such as negotiating a difficult family meeting, addressing existential distress, and managing refractory symptoms, would remain in the hands of HPM specialists.[73]

At present, CGSO fellowship trainees are reliant on the recommendations of surgical societies and the educational aims put forth by the Accreditation Council for Graduate Medical Education (ACGME) for PC curriculum content during fellowship training. This situation is due, in part, to the fact that PC training has not yet been incorporated into general surgery training—a prerequisite for matching into a CGSO fellowship—despite strong advocacy for its inclusion.[55,75] The ACGME—the governing body responsible for the accreditation of all US graduate medical programs—currently recommends that CGSO fellowship trainees be familiar with limited facets of PC, specifically that CGSO fellowship programs (1) educate trainees on when to make appropriate referrals for PC,[76] (2) perform palliative surgical procedures when appropriate,[77] and (3) have a knowledge of nonsurgical palliative treatments.[77] How training programs accomplish these aims and assess for competence is left to the discretion of individual programs.[78,79]

Surgical societal recommendations do not strongly differ from that of the ACGME's. In fact, the SSO has yet to release a statement on PC, likely because PC has already been embraced and advocated for by ASCO and is perceived as falling under ASCO's umbrella. ASCO's initial provisional clinical opinion recommending that PC be combined with standard oncology care early in the course of illness for any patient with metastatic cancer and/or high symptom burden was released in 2012.[80] In 2017, this clinical opinion was updated with 2 new recommendations: (1) early PC should be administered concomitantly with active treatment, and (2) providers should consider referring caregivers of patients with early or advanced cancer to PC services.[1] These recommendations in their entirety are significant and build on the 2005 10-point principles of PC statement released by the American College of Surgeons (ACS)—the largest organization of surgeons in the world.[81]

POOR COMMUNICATION AMONG PROVIDERS AND BETWEEN PROVIDERS AND PATIENTS ABOUT PALLIATIVE CARE

Communication—the most fundamental aspect of patient-provider relations—has long served as a barrier to equitable utilization of PC on several fronts.[11,45] PC is often either discussed very late in the clinical course of a patient with cancer,[82] not clearly explained to the patient,[11] or not discussed clearly or to a significant extent among providers who are caring for mutual patients.[11]

Recognizing that patients still consider health care providers to be the primary source for knowledge about PC[59] only serves to amplify the significance of communication in promoting equitable use of health care services. In a study by Zimmermann and colleagues, 48 patients and 23 caregivers were interviewed after completing a randomized controlled trial of early PC versus standard care for patients with advanced cancer.[46] The investigators observed that patients' perceptions of PC provoked fear and avoidance, which often originated from their interactions with health care providers.[46] These misperceptions eroded over the course of the study but highlight the power that preconceived attitudes, feelings, and beliefs can have and underscore the potential impact of provider interactions. The significance of provider communication was not lost on patients, as many pointed out PC could have been better framed and explained by health care professionals.[46]

In a separate study that examined whether African Americans were informed about hospice services by their health care providers, the investigators identified communication on the subject as significantly lacking. Contrary to Zimmerman and colleagues where patients were randomized to early PC versus standard care, Rhodes and colleagues retrospectively examined a cohort of 111 patients to see if PC was even discussed.[83] Their findings following 1578 interviews with the informants of the dece-dents revealed that most African Americans were not provided information regarding hospice services but that among those who were informed, many chose to enroll.[83] Although patients with cancer were more likely than others to be counseled about hos-pice,[83] this study makes clear that disparities in the quality of provided communication may be perpetuated by health care providers working with marginalized populations.

Causes for failed communication remain numerous. Some providers are not willing to encourage timely and appropriate utilization of PC due to potential family resistance and fear of being perceived as "giving up."[57] Others feel that the involvement of a PC team will lead to the miscommunication of prognostic information to patients and their families.[57] Ironically, many surgeons overrate the benefit of their own discussions with patients regarding prognosis as assessed by their colleagues.[84] Conversations regarding PC are not easy. Some providers, in fact, avoid having PC discussions due to the stress caused by being exposed to such stressful and traumatic patient life events.[85] It has even been postulated that some providers may avoid engaging PC services due to their own attitudes and fears about death.[86,87]

Deficits in communication, however, extend beyond patient-provider relationships; there are significant improvements needed in provider-provider communication. Le and colleagues conducted interviews with 28 clinicians in order to identify the feasi-bility of integrating PC early in the clinical course of patients with incurable lung can-cer.[12] They identified a need for effective communication among health care providers in the coordination of care patients received, especially when patients moved between hospital and home.[12] Information flow during these transitions seemed easily disrup-ted. Physicians from different teams are not always clear with each other about what has been communicated to mutual patients, making prioritization of next steps in care coordination difficult to discern.

FUTURE DIRECTIONS

As has been made clear in this article, inequities in access to and utilization of PC exist among patients with cancer. The causes are numerous and complex. Dismantling these barriers will require coordinated efforts.

To resolve current PC knowledge gaps, we should acknowledge current training deficits, determine the type of workforce we need, and implement effective PC training strategies. Having a trained workforce should foster more awareness of the practice, lead to a more informed public, and promote increased and equitable PC utilization. Leaders from organizations including ASCO, SSO, ACS, and HPM should consider meeting to agree on the roles of "PC Champions," especially given the increasing de-mand for HPM specialists. This coordinated effort, in turn, should lead to the develop-ment of an appropriate curriculum and method for evaluating competency.

Several PC training resources are available. There is one text resource for surgical trainees, titled "Surgical Palliative Care: A Resident's Guide."[88] Collaboratively pub-lished by the Cunniff-Dixon Foundation and the ACS in 2009, it is a robust resource that has been used by several groups as a framework for PC immersion training pro-grams and workshops.[89,90] There are also several Web sites that offer online curricula, which on completion are paired with certificates and/or continuing medical education/continuing education unit credits (eg, The Center to Advance Palliative Care, Harvard Medical School Center for Palliative Care).

PC training alone, however, will not resolve current barriers if members of our work-force cannot effectively communicate among themselves and with our patients.[8,12] There are several programs that provide training in communication (eg, VitalTalk,

The Center to Advance Palliative Care). Consideration should also be given to pairing this training with cultural competency training,[6,91] given the culturally diverse populations we treat and our nation's legacy of systemic racism. Determining effective strategies for improving intergroup communication is an additional need that may require some innovation, but as the COVID-19 pandemic has shown us through our use of video visits and video tumor boards, communication can evolve when necessary.

Dismantling current barriers for racial and ethnic minorities is likely to prove more challenging, given the structural barriers these groups have long faced in the United States. Increasing the diversity in the medical workforce is one strategy.[92] A workforce trained in communication and PC will also undoubtedly help, but additional factors may need to be addressed. It is hoped that ongoing studies such as EQUAL APC[43] will elucidate some; additional research conducted with minority populations and consistent reporting of race should shed light on others. Notably, of the 18 trials cited in the 2012 and 2017 ASCO clinical statements on early integration of PC, only one-third reported racial and ethnic minority representation.[93] The importance of this oversight cannot be overstated. Different causes require different interventions. If differences in equitable access to PC are the result of patient preferences, then we should consider developing appropriate educational initiatives.

SUMMARY

Unfortunately, PC remains inequitably accessible, underutilized, and is still too often introduced late in the care of patients receiving surgical intervention,[4] despite evidence that PC has the potential to reduce health care utilization and improve ACP without affecting mortality.[5] As a community of surgeons who care for patients with cancer, we know all too well the inordinate physical, psychosocial, and spiritual tolls that undertreated pain and other end-of-life concerns can take on patients and their families. Fortunately, and as has been highlighted here, the numerous and complex barriers to equitable PC utilization among patients with cancer can be dismantled, and optimizing quality of life without disrupting active cancer treatment can be achieved. Progress in this arena will require coordinated efforts at the level of providers, professional organizations, and policymakers. Research is needed to inform these efforts to provide the right care at the right time equitably.

DISCLOSURE

The authors have nothing to disclose.

REFERENCES

1. Ferrell BR, Temel JS, Temin S, et al. Integration of Palliative Care Into Standard Oncology Care: American Society of Clinical Oncology Clinical Practice Guideline Update. J Clin Oncol 2017;35(1):96–112.
2. Clark D. From margins to centre: a review of the history of palliative care in cancer. Lancet Oncol 2007;8(5):430–8.
3. Sepulveda C, Marlin A, Yoshida T, et al. Palliative Care: the World Health Organization's global perspective. J Pain Symptom Manage 2002;24(2):91–6.
4. Sarradon-Eck A, Besle S, Troian J, et al. Understanding the Barriers to Introducing Early Palliative Care for Patients with Advanced Cancer: A Qualitative Study. J Palliat Med 2019;22(5):508–16.
5. Lilley EJ, Khan KT, Johnston FM, et al. Palliative Care Interventions for Surgical Patients: A Systematic Review. JAMA Surg 2016;151(2):172–83.

6. Griggs JJ. Disparities in Palliative Care in Patients With Cancer. J Clin Oncol 2020;38(9):974–9.

7. Institute of Medicine (US) Committee on Understanding and Eliminating Racial and Ethnic Disparities in Health Care. Unequal Treatment: Confronting Racial and Ethnic Disparities in Health Care. Smedley BD, Stith AY, Nelson AR, editors. Washington (DC): National Academies Press (US); 2003.

8. Fahy BN. Introduction: Role of palliative care for the surgical patient. J Surg Oncol 2019;120(1):5–9.

9. Kelley AS, Morrison RS. Palliative Care for the Seriously Ill. N Engl J Med 2015; 373(8):747–55.

10. Kamal AH, Bull JH, Swetz KM, et al. Future of the Palliative Care Workforce: Preview to an Impending Crisis. Am J Med 2017;130(2):113–4.

11. Suwanabol PA, Kanters AE, Reichstein AC, et al. Characterizing the Role of U.S. Surgeons in the Provision of Palliative Care: A Systematic Review and Mixed-Methods Meta-Synthesis. J Pain Symptom Manage 2018;55(4):1196–215.e5.

12. Le BH, Mileshkin L, Doan K, et al. Acceptability of early integration of palliative care in patients with incurable lung cancer. J Palliat Med 2014;17(5):553–8.

13. Shen MJ, Wellman JD. Evidence of palliative care stigma: The role of negative stereotypes in preventing willingness to use palliative care. Palliat Support Care 2019;17(4):374–80.

14. Haviland K, Burrows Walters C, Newman S. Barriers to palliative care in sexual and gender minority patients with cancer: A scoping review of the literature. Health Soc Care Community 2020;29(2):305–18.

15. Adam E, Sleeman KE, Brearley S, et al. The palliative care needs of adults with intellectual disabilities and their access to palliative care services: A systematic review. Palliat Med 2020;34(8):1006–18.

16. Davies B, Sehring SA, Partridge JC, et al. Barriers to palliative care for children: perceptions of pediatric health care providers. Pediatrics 2008;121(2):282–8.

17. Parajuli J, Tark A, Jao YL, et al. Barriers to palliative and hospice care utilization in older adults with cancer: A systematic review. J Geriatr Oncol 2020;11(1):8–16.

18. Oncology SoS. Society of Surgical Oncology Statement on Racism, Diversity and Cancer Care. 2020. Available at: https://www.surgonc.org/about-sso/society-of-surgical-oncology-statement-on-racism-diversity-and-cancer-care/.   Accessed February 1, 2021.

19. Reyes-Gibby CC, Anderson KO, Shete S, et al. Early referral to supportive care specialists for symptom burden in lung cancer patients: a comparison of non-Hispanic whites, Hispanics, and non-Hispanic blacks. Cancer 2012;118(3): 856–63.

20. Sanders JJ, Robinson MT, Block SD. Factors Impacting Advance Care Planning among African Americans: Results of a Systematic Integrated Review. J Palliat Med 2016;19(2):202–27.

21. Smith AK, Earle CC, McCarthy EP. Racial and ethnic differences in end-of-life care in fee-for-service Medicare beneficiaries with advanced cancer. J Am Geriatr Soc 2009;57(1):153–8.

22. Fishman J, O'Dwyer P, Lu HL, et al. Race, treatment preferences, and hospice enrollment: eligibility criteria may exclude patients with the greatest needs for care. Cancer 2009;115(3):689–97.

23. Cohen LL. Racial/ethnic disparities in hospice care: a systematic review. J Palliat Med 2008;11(5):763–8.

24. Ornstein KA, Roth DL, Huang J, et al. Evaluation of Racial Disparities in Hospice Use and End-of-Life Treatment Intensity in the REGARDS Cohort. JAMA Netw Open 2020;3(8):e2014639.
25. Ingersoll LT, Alexander SC, Priest J, et al. Racial/ethnic differences in prognosis communication during initial inpatient palliative care consultations among people with advanced cancer. Patient Educ Couns 2019;102(6):1098–103.
26. Gramling R, Gajary-Coots E, Cimino J, et al. Palliative Care Clinician Overestimation of Survival in Advanced Cancer: Disparities and Association With End-of-Life Care. J Pain Symptom Manage 2019;57(2):233–40.
27. Loggers ET, Maciejewski PK, Paulk E, et al. Racial differences in predictors of intensive end-of-life care in patients with advanced cancer. J Clin Oncol 2009; 27(33):5559–64.
28. Rosenzweig MQ, Wiehagen T, Brufsky A, et al. Challenges of illness in metastatic breast cancer: a low-income African American perspective. Palliat Support Care 2009;7(2):143–52.
29. Barnato AE, Anthony DL, Skinner J, et al. Racial and ethnic differences in preferences for end-of-life treatment. J Gen Intern Med 2009;24(6):695–701.
30. Smith AK, Davis RB, Krakauer EL. Differences in the quality of the patient-physician relationship among terminally ill African-American and white patients: impact on advance care planning and treatment preferences. J Gen Intern Med 2007;22(11):1579–82.
31. Smith AK, McCarthy EP, Paulk E, et al. Racial and ethnic differences in advance care planning among patients with cancer: impact of terminal illness acknowledgment, religiousness, and treatment preferences. J Clin Oncol 2008;26(25): 4131–7.
32. Harrison KL, Adrion ER, Ritchie CS, et al. Low Completion and Disparities in Advance Care Planning Activities Among Older Medicare Beneficiaries. JAMA Intern Med 2016;176(12):1872–5.
33. Ranganathan A, Gunnarsson O, Casarett D. Palliative care and advance care planning for patients with advanced malignancies. Ann Palliat Med 2014;3(3): 144–9.
34. National Comprehensive Cancer Network. Palliative Care (Version 2.2021). Available at: https://www.nccn.org/professionals/physician_gls/PDF/palliative.pdf. Accessed February 17, 2021.
35. Phipps E, True G, Harris D, et al. Approaching the end of life: attitudes, preferences, and behaviors of African-American and white patients and their family caregivers. J Clin Oncol 2003;21(3):549–54.
36. Crawley LM. Palliative care in African American communities. J Palliat Med 2002; 5(5):775–9.
37. Juckett G. Cross-cultural medicine. Am Fam Physician 2005;72(11):2267–74.
38. Laury ER, MacKenzie-Greenle M, Meghani S. Advance Care Planning Outcomes in African Americans: An Empirical Look at the Trust Variable. J Palliat Med 2019; 22(4):442–51.
39. Gamble VN. Under the shadow of Tuskegee: African Americans and health care. Am J Public Health 1997;87(11):1773–8.
40. Payne R. Improving Palliative Care for African-American & Other Minority Patients. Oncol Times 2002;24(5):2–4.
41. True G, Phipps EJ, Braitman LE, et al. Treatment preferences and advance care planning at end of life: the role of ethnicity and spiritual coping in cancer patients. Ann Behav Med 2005;30(2):174–9.

42. Johnson J, Hayden T, True J, et al. The Impact of Faith Beliefs on Perceptions of End-of-Life Care and Decision Making among African American Church Members. J Palliat Med 2016;19(2):143–8.

43. Ejem DB, Barrett N, Rhodes RL, et al. Reducing Disparities in the Quality of Palliative Care for Older African Americans through Improved Advance Care Planning: Study Design and Protocol. J Palliat Med 2019;22(S1):90–100.

44. den Herder-van der Eerden M, Ewert B, Hodiamont F, et al. Towards accessible integrated palliative care: Perspectives of leaders from seven European countries on facilitators, barriers and recommendations for improvement. J Integr Care (Brighton) 2017;25(3):222–32.

45. Suwanabol PA, Reichstein AC, Suzer-Gurtekin ZT, et al. Surgeons' Perceived Barriers to Palliative and End-of-Life Care: A Mixed Methods Study of a Surgical Society. J Palliat Med 2018;21(6):780–8.

46. Zimmermann C, Swami N, Krzyzanowska M, et al. Perceptions of palliative care among patients with advanced cancer and their caregivers. CMAJ 2016;188(10): E217–27.

47. Fadul N, Elsayem A, Palmer JL, et al. Supportive versus palliative care: what's in a name?: a survey of medical oncologists and midlevel providers at a comprehensive cancer center. Cancer 2009;115(9):2013–21.

48. Johnson KS. Racial and ethnic disparities in palliative care. J Palliat Med 2013; 16(11):1329–34.

49. Born W, Greiner KA, Sylvia E, et al. Knowledge, attitudes, and beliefs about end-of-life care among inner-city African Americans and Latinos. J Palliat Med 2004; 7(2):247–56.

50. Johnson KS, Kuchibhatla M, Tulsky JA. Racial differences in self-reported exposure to information about hospice care. J Palliat Med 2009;12(10):921–7.

51. Wasserman J, Palmer RC, Gomez MM, et al. Advancing Health Services Research to Eliminate Health Care Disparities. Am J Public Health 2019; 109(S1):S64–9.

52. Rajdev K, Loghmanieh N, Farberov MA, et al. Are Health-Care Providers Well Prepared in Providing Optimal End-of-Life Care to Critically Ill Patients? A Cross-Sectional Study at a Tertiary Care Hospital in the United States. J Intensive Care Med 2020;35(10):1080–94.

53. Rodriguez R, Marr L, Rajput A, et al. Utilization of palliative care consultation service by surgical services. Ann Palliat Med 2015;4(4):194–9.

54. Scally CP, Robinson K, Blumenthaler AN, et al. Identifying Core Principles of Palliative Care Consultation in Surgical Patients and Potential Knowledge Gaps for Surgeons. J Am Coll Surg 2020;231(1):179–85.

55. Bateni SB, Canter RJ, Meyers FJ, et al. Palliative care training and decision-making for patients with advanced cancer: a comparison of surgeons and medical physicians. Surgery 2018. https://doi.org/10.1016/j.surg.2018.01.021.

56. Evans BA, Turner MC, Gloria JN, et al. Palliative Care Consultation Is Underutilized in Critically Ill General Surgery Patients. Am J Hosp Palliat Care 2020; 37(2):149–53.

57. Karlekar M, Collier B, Parish A, et al. Utilization and determinants of palliative care in the trauma intensive care unit: results of a national survey. Palliat Med 2014; 28(8):1062–8.

58. Sorensen A, Wentlandt K, Le LW, et al. Practices and opinions of specialized palliative care physicians regarding early palliative care in oncology. Support Care Cancer 2020;28(2):877–85.

59. Huo J, Hong YR, Grewal R, et al. Knowledge of Palliative Care Among American Adults: 2018 Health Information National Trends Survey. J Pain Symptom Manage 2019;58(1):39–47 e33.

60. Amini A, Miura JT, Larrieux G, et al. Palliative care training in surgical oncology and hepatobiliary fellowships: a national survey of the fellows. Ann Surg Oncol 2015;22(6):1761–7.

61. Galante JM, Bowles TL, Khatri VP, et al. Experience and attitudes of surgeons toward palliation in cancer. Arch Surg 2005;140(9):873–8 [discussion: 878–80].

62. Medicine AAoHaP. Workforce Data and Reports. 2019. Available at: http://aahpm.org/career/workforce-study. Accessed July 28, 2020.

63. Cameron J, Cameron A. Current surgical therapy. 13th edition. Philadelphia, PA: Elsevier; 2019.

64. Brunicardi F, Anderson D, Billiar T, et al. Schwartz's principles of surgery. 11th edition. New York, NY: McGraw-Hill Education; 2019.

65. Townsend C, Beauchamp R, Evers B, et al. Sabiston textbook of surgery - the biological basis of modern surgical practice. 20th edition. Philadelphia, PA: Elsevier; 2016.

66. Mulholland M, Lillemoe K, Doherty G, et al. Greenfield's surgery - scientific principles and practice. Philadelphia, PA: Wolters Kluwer Health; 2016.

67. Fischer J, Jones D, Pomposelli F, et al. Fischer's mastery of surgery. Philadelphia, PA: Lippincott Williams & Wilkins; 2018.

68. Morita S, Balch C, Klimberg V, et al. Textbook of complex general surgical oncology. 1st edition. New York, NY: The McGraw-Hill Companies, Inc; 2018.

69. Thomas RA, Curley B, Wen S, et al. Palliative Care Training during Fellowship: A National Survey of U.S. Hematology and Oncology Fellows. J Palliat Med 2015; 18(9):747–51.

70. Wong A, Reddy A, Williams JL, et al. ReCAP: Attitudes, Beliefs, and Awareness of Graduate Medical Education Trainees Regarding Palliative Care at a Comprehensive Cancer Center. J Oncol Pract 2016;12(2):149–50, e127-137.

71. Morin L, Aubry R, Frova L, et al. Estimating the need for palliative care at the population level: A cross-national study in 12 countries. Palliat Med 2017;31(6): 526–36.

72. Lupu D, American Academy of H, Palliative Medicine Workforce Task F. Estimate of current hospice and palliative medicine physician workforce shortage. J Pain Symptom Manage 2010;40(6):899–911.

73. Quill TE, Abernethy AP. Generalist plus specialist palliative care–creating a more sustainable model. N Engl J Med 2013;368(13):1173–5.

74. Kamal AH, Bowman B, Ritchie CS. Identifying Palliative Care Champions to Promote High-Quality Care to Those with Serious Illness. J Am Geriatr Soc 2019; 67(S2):S461–7.

75. Sigman M, Miller P. Practicing primary palliative care: A call to action. Bull Am Coll Surg 2019;104(11):13–21.

76. Accreditation Council for Graduate Medical Education. The Complex General Surgical Oncology Milestone Project. 2014. Available at: http://www.acgme.org/Portals/0/PDFs/Milestones/CGSO.pdf. Accessed July 28, 2020.

77. Education ACfGM. ACGME Program Requirements for Graduate Medical Education in Complex General Surgical Oncology. 2020. Available at: https://www.acgme.org/Portals/0/PFAssets/ProgramResources/446_ComplexGeneralSurgicalOncology_2020_TCC.pdf?ver=2020-02-17-090323-063. Accessed July 28, 2020.

78. Badgwell B. Will Palliative Care Ever Be Cool? Ann Surg Oncol 2018;25(7): 1799–800.
79. Robbins JR, Kilari D, Johnston F. Palliative care education for oncologists: how are we doing? Ann Palliat Med 2019;8(4):364–71.
80. Smith TJ, Temin S, Alesi ER, et al. American Society of Clinical Oncology provisional clinical opinion: the integration of palliative care into standard oncology care. J Clin Oncol 2012;30(8):880–7.
81. Task Force on Surgical Palliative c, Committee on E. Statement of principles of palliative care. Bull Am Coll Surg 2005;90(8):34–5.
82. Mack JW, Cronin A, Taback N, et al. End-of-life care discussions among patients with advanced cancer: a cohort study. Ann Intern Med 2012;156(3):204–10.
83. Rhodes RL, Teno JM, Welch LC. Access to hospice for African Americans: are they informed about the option of hospice? J Palliat Med 2006;9(2):268–72.
84. Aslakson RA, Wyskiel R, Shaeffer D, et al. Surgical intensive care unit clinician estimates of the adequacy of communication regarding patient prognosis. Crit Care 2010;14(6):R218.
85. Granek L, Nakash O, Cohen M, et al. Oncologists' communication about end of life: the relationship among secondary traumatic stress, compassion satisfaction, and approach and avoidance communication. Psychooncology 2017;26(11): 1980–6.
86. Cripe L, Frankel RM. Understanding what influences oncology clinicians' communicating with dying patients: Awareness of one's own mortality may be one key. Patient Educ Couns 2016;99(3):307–9.
87. Draper EJ, Hillen MA, Moors M, et al. Relationship between physicians' death anxiety and medical communication and decision-making: A systematic review. Patient Educ Couns 2019;102(2):266–74.
88. Dunn GP, Martensen R, Weissman D, editors. Surgical palliative care: a Resident's Guide. Chicago: American College of Surgeons; 2009.
89. Pernar LI, Peyre SE, Smink DS, et al. Feasibility and impact of a case-based palliative care workshop for general surgery residents. J Am Coll Surg 2012;214(2): 231–6.
90. Raoof M, O'Neill L, Neumayer L, et al. Prospective evaluation of surgical palliative care immersion training for general surgery residents. Am J Surg 2017;214(2): 378–83.
91. Rhodes RL, Batchelor K, Lee SC, et al. Barriers to end-of-life care for African Americans from the providers' perspective: opportunity for intervention development. Am J Hosp Palliat Care 2015;32(2):137–43.
92. Stanford FC. The Importance of Diversity and Inclusion in the Healthcare Workforce. J Natl Med Assoc 2020;112(3):247–9.
93. Pirl WF, Saez-Flores E, Schlumbrecht M, et al. Race and Ethnicity in the Evidence for Integrating Palliative Care Into Oncology. J Oncol Pract 2018;14(6):e346–56.

Disparities in Creating a Diverse Surgical Oncology Physician Workforce

Just a Leaky Pipeline?

Callisia N. Clarke, MD, MS

KEYWORDS

- Underrepresented minority in medicine • URM • Physician workforce diversity
- Cancer disparities • Surgical oncology

KEY POINTS

- Disparate cancer outcomes are projected to increase as the United States (US) population becomes more racially and ethnically diverse.
- There is a critical shortage of physicians who are underrepresented in medicine (URM); this paucity is especially profound in oncology subspecialties and within surgical oncology in particular.
- The proportion of URM students entering medical school, surgical residency, and complex general surgical oncology fellowships significantly decreases at each level, resulting in a precariously empty and continuously leaking pipeline.
- URM faculty recruitment, retention, and advancement in surgical oncology are hindered by implicit bias and microaggressions, resulting in attrition.

INTRODUCTION

The Unites States (US) is diversifying faster than predicted, so much so that the US Census Bureau predicts that by 2045, White Americans will no longer be in the majority.[1] As the proportion of racial and ethnic minorities increases in our aging population, so will the total projected cancer incidence.[2] Minorities are particularly vulnerable to suboptimal cancer care and disparate cancer outcomes for a variety of reasons. Ethnic and racial minorities are largely underrepresented in cancer clinical trials and are less likely to receive standard-of-care cancer treatments.[3] As the demographic shifts in our population continue, the potential for widening an already-concerning gap in cancer outcomes between minority populations when compared with their White counterparts is a substantial threat to our health care system. From 2010 to 2030, total cancer incidence in the US is projected to increase by approximately

Division of Surgical Oncology, 8701 West Watertown Plank Road, Milwaukee, WI 53226, USA
E-mail address: cnclarke@mcw.edu

Surg Oncol Clin N Am 31 (2022) 21–27
https://doi.org/10.1016/j.soc.2021.07.004
1055-3207/22/© 2021 Elsevier Inc. All rights reserved.

45% to 2.3 million.[2] This increase is largely driven by an anticipated 99% increase in cancer diagnoses in minority populations compared with a 31% increase for Whites.[2] From 2010 to 2030, the percentage of US minorities with a cancer diagnosis is expected to increase from 21% to 28%. As such, every effort to close the cancer care gap must be prioritized to improve oncologic outcomes and access for minorities.

Unfortunately, the diversity of our physician workforce has not kept pace with the diversity of the patient populations we serve. In 2003, the Association of American Medical Colleges (AAMC) acknowledged this burgeoning reality and adopted the term "underrepresented in medicine (URM)," defined as racial and ethnic populations represented at lower rates in the medical profession than the general US population. Racial and ethnic minorities are more likely to provide care for medically underserved communities than their White counterparts, and patients of color are more likely to seek out physicians of color to provide their care.[4–6] The impact of physician race and gender on receipt of preventative services and patient satisfaction has also been widely documented.[7,8] For these reasons, creating and maintaining a diverse physician workforce is critical to any effort aimed at eliminating health care disparities and improving health equity overall.

In 2019, 60.1% of the US population identified as White, 18.5% Hispanic, 12.5% Black, 5.8% Asian, 2.2% other, and 0.7% American Indian/Alaska Native.[1] During the same year, AAMC US physician workforce data demonstrated that Hispanics, Blacks, and Native Americans remain grossly underrepresented in medicine, accounting for only 5.8%, 5.0%, and 0.3% of practicing physicians, respectively.[9] Now, more than ever, it has become urgent that the oncology workforce reflect the underlying population of patients with cancer it serves. However, we continue to struggle to recruit and retain racial and ethnic minorities to oncology subspecialties, resulting in even poorer physician diversity than medicine overall.[10]

The field of surgical oncology in particular faces a steep challenge in attaining the necessary physician diversity to meet our patients' needs. Low racial and ethnic diversity in surgery is persistent. Only 13.6% of students matriculating into medical school are URM with Blacks accounting for only 7.1% and Hispanics accounting for 6.2% of matriculating medical students in 2018.[9] Even fewer URM students enter general surgery residencies. Of all general surgery trainees in 2020, only 5.3% identified as Black, 8.1% as Hispanic/Latino, 0.8% American Indian, and 0.3% Pacific Islander.[11] More alarmingly, of all active Complex General Surgical Oncology fellows in academic year 2019 to 2020, 69.4% were White, 5.6% Hispanic/Latino, and only 1.9% Black or African American.[11] As it relates to creating a diverse surgical oncology physician workforce, the pipeline in essentially empty.

Academic institutions carry the brunt of the responsibility in working to correct these issues. Academic medicine is a complex "system that produces the human capital, including the physicians who care for the patients and the educators who train those physicians."[12] They are the gate keepers that decide who gets the "privilege" of entry into medical school, residencies, and fellowships. If we are to really address the lack of racial and ethnic diversity in surgical oncology, we must start with these institutions first. After completing surgical training, women and minorities are less likely to enter academic practices and when they do, they are often faced with limited opportunities for advancement when compared with their White male colleagues.[13,14] Black surgeons are less likely to be promoted from assistant professor to associate professor than any other ethnic group.[15] These measurable disparities and other intangible biases contribute to high rates of attrition for women and URM faculty, thereby compounding the lack of diversity in academic surgical oncology. Simply put, for the URM surgeons within the system, an already near-empty pipeline is *also* leaky.

INCREASING DIVERSITY IN SURGICAL ONCOLOGY

Increasing racial and ethnic diversity in the surgical oncology physician workforce requires intentionality and commitment. Successful efforts will necessitate the development of coordinated, well-supported programs of longer duration that target multiple components necessary to increase the pool of potential applicants and enhance the recruitment and retention of these talented individuals into surgical oncology. These programs require time and investment and must adapt and mature to yield consistent results.

Increasing the Pipeline into General Surgery and Surgical Oncology Training Programs

After the AAMC defined URM and addressed the need for improved racial and ethnic diversity in the physician workforce, significant formalized efforts have been directed at increasing the pipeline of women and URM students applying to medical schools. These efforts have had modest benefits to date as the percentage of URMs applying to medical school has remained essentially unchanged over the past decade. For URM medical students applying to residencies, surgery is a daunting challenge. Attrition in general surgery residency remains high, and attrition that occurs in the later years is the most worrisome. Unpublished data (William A. McDade; 2020) suggest that Black general surgery residents are almost twenty times more likely to be dismissed from surgery residency than their White counterparts. In one study, Hispanic trainees were more likely to leave before completing general surgery residency with an attrition rate of 21.1% versus 12.4% than non-Hispanic residents.[14] These issues of attrition do not happen in isolation. In a recent comprehensive resident survey, Black general surgery residents had a 20.9 times higher likelihood of experiencing racial discrimination throughout their training.[16] Hispanic and Asian residents also experienced significant discrimination, though at lower rates with odds ratios of 2.62 and 6.29 ($P<.001$), respectively.[16] These incidents assail the mental health of URM trainees and directly impact their willingness to pursue further subspecialty training in fields including complex general surgical oncology. Academic residency programs must adopt a zero-tolerance policy for anyone witnessing or experiencing toxic behaviors, discrimination, or harassment, and the most vulnerable of our residents must be empowered to speak up without risk of retaliation. Complex General Surgical Oncology fellowship programs must also prioritize recruitment of URM trainees to the field. The implementation of visiting rotations for URM candidates has been proven effective, and increased awareness has prompted many national societies to create targeted programs to address URM trainee recruitment to oncology. Increased faculty diversity—especially at the program-director level and among those conducting interviews and small-group social events for URM applicants and faculty—have been effective tools used in other specialties and should be strongly encouraged for all training programs.[17]

Increasing Underrepresented in Medicine Surgical Oncology Faculty Recruitment and Retention

Recruitment and hiring practices in academic surgery are rarely discussed. It is widely accepted that intentional recruitment practices directly influence diversity efforts. However, there are no established standards or best practices widely used to enhance recruitment of diverse surgical faculty. Reliance on trusted networks is a strategy widely used by most institutions when hiring in academia, but this targeted recruitment strategy often results in a small, homogenous applicant pool and may further limit the number of URM physicians who ultimately apply for, and gain entry into, surgical faculty positions. Furthermore, implicit bias plays a role in recruitment and hiring processes. When evaluating curricula vitae (CVs), women and minorities are more likely to have their technical skills and academic achievements questioned despite objective data to the contrary.[18,19] In studies of equivalent fictitious resumes, CVs of perceived African American candidates were rated negatively, while those of Asian American candidates were rated more positively despite similar qualifications.[20]

Recruitment of high-performing URM surgical oncology faculty is certainly possible when diversity is a central tenet within departments of surgery. Dossett and colleagues[21] describe the implementation of inclusive surgical faculty recruitment strategies at their institution, and several recruitment practices they used warrant special consideration. First, all individuals participating in recruitment activities underwent mandatory training addressing implicit bias. Each recruitment team had diverse membership, and all positions were broadly advertised through traditional and nontraditional venues, specifically targeting organizations focused on URM physicians. They implemented a standardized interview, evaluation, and scoring protocol to minimize subjectivity and bias. Although the process is certainly more time- and resource-intensive, the desired outcome of increased diversity in the applicant pool and new surgical faculty hires was achieved.[21]

Enhanced retention practices for URM surgical oncology faculty must also accompany strategies to improve recruitment. Academic surgery continues to experience high rates of bullying, sexual harassment, and microaggression that undermine the health and safety of workplace environments and impact faculty wellness as well as patient safety.[22] The negative impact of these experiences on URM faculty promotion and advancement cannot be easily measured but is likely to be both pervasive and profound. Racial and ethnic minorities are more likely to report experiencing conscious and unconscious bias from colleagues, patients, and students.[23,24] These experiences result in disparate faculty evaluation and patient satisfaction scores that negatively impact determination of readiness for promotion or suitability for leadership. Although there are limited data on attrition rates in surgical oncology specifically, within academic surgery as a whole, these negative interactions and the concomitantly unfavorable evaluations they engender represent just some of the many factors that contribute to lower compensation, low rates of retention, and slower pace of promotion among faculty of color.[15,25] Department leaders and promotion committees must be aware of these patterns to avoid unintentionally perpetuating existing problems, and they must work to create inclusive work environments free of harassment or discrimination.

Creating Opportunities for Underrepresented in Medicine Advancement and Promotion

Attempts to improve racial and ethnic diversity among surgical oncologists must not only include effective recruitment strategies but also include professional development opportunities that will lead to academic success, promotion, and retention. Over the past 10 years, there has been an approximately 15% to 20% decrease in the proportion of Black associate professors of surgery and a 3% decrease in the proportion of Black full professors of surgery.[26] The proportion of Hispanic associate and full professors of surgery has increased over the same time period, whereas Hispanics remain significantly underrepresented, accounting for only 6% of all surgical faculty members when compared with 18% of the general population.[26–28] Because academic rank contributes significantly to compensation, inequities in promotion perpetuate lower salary ranges for URM faculty than for their peers and likely increase rates of attrition.[29]

Academic institutions, professional societies, and governing bodies have more recently embraced the value of formalized leadership development programs for URM physicians. In academic surgery, women, Blacks, Hispanics, and Asian Americans remain significantly underrepresented in leadership.[30] Asian Americans are overrepresented in medicine when compared with the US population but are less likely to be promoted to leadership positions in surgery. Similarly, despite increasing representation in academic surgery, there continues to be a paucity of women in positions of leadership.[30] These data negate the argument that attaining a diverse surgical leadership is simply a function of creating a pipeline. A recent publication analyzing representation in leadership at the National Cancer Institute-Designated Cancer Centers demonstrated that among the 63 cancer centers with 856 leadership team members evaluated, 82.2% of cancer center leaders were White, 3.5% Black, 3.8% Hispanic, and 11% Asian.[31] More alarmingly, 23 NCI cancer centers (36.5%) did not have any Black or Hispanic representation in leadership and 8 cancer centers (12.7%) had all-White leadership teams.[31] These data point to a set of deeply entrenched barriers that favor the promotion of White physicians to leadership while inhibiting similar opportunities for minorities and highlight the critical need for intentional mentorship and sponsorship for URM faculty advancement into oncology leadership. Importantly, these initiatives must be developed with the input of minority faculty; must align with departmental, cancer center, and institutional goals; and are most effective when created with concrete financial support and resources from institutional leaders.

SUMMARY

Attaining equity in cancer outcomes is contingent on creating and maintaining a diverse physician workforce that reflects the communities we serve. In surgical oncology, the pipeline is both empty and leaky. Fewer URM medical students enter general surgery residencies, and even fewer pursue additional training in surgical oncology. Representation of URM surgeons in academic surgical oncology continues to lag and disparities in promotion and leadership advancement remain. To address these workforce gaps, institutions must intentionally recruit diverse surgical residents, fellows, and faculty members. Departments must achieve and maintain environments that embrace diversity and promote inclusivity, prioritize transparency in promotion and compensation, and champion career and leadership development programs that promote URM faculty to positions in leadership. Only then can we, as surgical oncologists, realistically hope to provide universally high-quality cancer care to minority patients and to mitigate the disparities in cancer screening, prevention, diagnosis, and treatment that continue to be observed in these groups.

DISCLOSURE

Research reported in this publication was supported by the National Institute of Diabetes and Digestive and Kidney Diseases of the National Institutes of Health under award number R01 DK052913-21S1.

REFERENCES

1. Population Data. 2020. Available at: https://usafacts.org/data/topics/people-society/population-and-demographics/population-data/population/#chart-114185-1. Accessed June 1, 2021.

2. Smith BD, Smith GL, Hurria A, et al. Future of cancer incidence in the United States: burdens upon an aging, changing nation. J Clin Oncol 2009;27(17): 2758–65.
3. Gross CP, Smith BD, Wolf E, et al. Racial disparities in cancer therapy: did the gap narrow between 1992 and 2002? Cancer 2008;112(4):900–8.
4. Xu G, Fields SK, Laine C, et al. The relationship between the race/ethnicity of generalist physicians and their care for underserved populations. Am J Public Health 1997;87(5):817–22.
5. Komaromy M, Grumbach K, Drake M, et al. The role of Black and Hispanic physicians in providing health care for underserved populations. N Engl J Med 1996; 334(20):1305–10.
6. Saha S, Komaromy M, Koepsell TD, et al. Patient-physician racial concordance and the perceived quality and use of health care. Arch Intern Med 1999; 159(9):997–1004.
7. Henderson JT, Weisman CS. Physician Gender Effects on Preventive Screening and Counseling: An Analysis of Male and Female Patients' Health Care Experiences. Med Care 2001;39(12):1281–92.
8. Schmittdiel J, Grumbach K, Selby JV, et al. Effect of physician and patient gender concordance on patient satisfaction and preventive care practices. J Gen Intern Med 2000;15(11):761–9.
9. Association of American Medical Colleges (2019). Diversity in Medicine: Facts and Figures 2019. 2019. Available at: https://www.aamc.org/data-reports/workforce/interactive-data/figure-18-percentage-all-active-physicians-race/ethnicity-2018. Accessed June 1, 2021.
10. American Society of Clinical. The State of Cancer Care in America, 2017: A Report by the American Society of Clinical Oncology. J Oncol Pract 2017;13(4): e353–94.
11. Association of American Medical Colleges (2020). Report on Residents. 2020. Available at: https://www.aamc.org/data-reports/students-residents/interactive-data/report-residents/2020/table-b5-md-residents-race-ethnicity-and-specialty. Accessed June 1, 2021.
12. Sanchez JP, Castillo-Page L, Spencer DJ, et al. Commentary: the building the next generation of academic physicians initiative: engaging medical students and residents. Acad Med 2011;86(8):928–31.
13. Abelson JS, Chartrand G, Moo TA, et al. The climb to break the glass ceiling in surgery: trends in women progressing from medical school to surgical training and academic leadership from 1994 to 2015. Am J Surg 2016;212(4):566.e1.
14. Yeo HL, Abelson JS, Symer MM, et al. Association of Time to Attrition in Surgical Residency With Individual Resident and Programmatic Factors. JAMA Surg 2018; 153(6):511–7.
15. Abelson JS, Wong NZ, Symer M, et al. Racial and ethnic disparities in promotion and retention of academic surgeons. Am J Surg 2018;216(4):678–82.
16. Yuce TK, Turner PL, Glass C, et al. National Evaluation of Racial/Ethnic Discrimination in US Surgical Residency Programs. JAMA Surg 2020;155(6):526–8.
17. Lewis T, Tolbert J, Jones BL. Increasing Resident Racial and Ethnic Diversity through Targeted Recruitment Efforts. J Pediatr 2020;216:4–6.
18. Putnam MD, Adams JE, Lender P, et al. Examination of Skill Acquisition and Grader Bias in a Distal Radius Fracture Fixation Model. J Surg Educ 2018; 75(5):1299–308.

19. Steinpreis RE, Anders KA, Ritzke D. The Impact of Gender on the Review of the Curricula Vitae of Job Applicants and Tenure Candidates: A National Empirical Study. Sex Roles 1999;41(7):509–28.
20. King EB, Mendoza SA, Madera JM, et al. What's in a Name? A Multiracial Investigation of the Role of Occupational Stereotypes in Selection Decisions. J Appl Social Pyschol 2006;36(5):1145–59.
21. Dossett LA, Mulholland MW, Newman EA. Building High-Performing Teams in Academic Surgery: The Opportunities and Challenges of Inclusive Recruitment Strategies. Acad Med 2019;94(8):1142–5.
22. Hu YY, Ellis RJ, Hewitt DB, et al. Discrimination, Abuse, Harassment, and Burnout in Surgical Residency Training. N Engl J Med 2019;381(18):1741–52.
23. Price EG, Gozu A, Kern DE, et al. The role of cultural diversity climate in recruitment, promotion, and retention of faculty in academic medicine. J Gen Intern Med 2005;20(7):565–71.
24. Peterson NB, Friedman RH, Ash AS, et al. Faculty self-reported experience with racial and ethnic discrimination in academic medicine. J Gen Intern Med 2004; 19(3):259–65.
25. Hoops HE, Brasel KJ, Dewey E, et al. Analysis of Gender-based Differences in Surgery Faculty Compensation, Promotion, and Retention: Establishing Equity. Ann Surg 2018;268(3):479–87.
26. Abelson JS, Symer MM, Yeo HL, et al. Surgical time out: Our counts are still short on racial diversity in academic surgery. Am J Surg 2018;215(4):542–8.
27. Unites States Census Bureau. 2019. Available at: https://www.census.gov/quickfacts/fact/table/US/PST045219#PST045219. Accessed June 1, 2021.
28. AAMC Diversity in Medicine: Facts and Figures 2019. 2019. Available at: https://www.aamc.org/data-reports/workforce/report/diversity-medicine-facts-and-figures-2019. Accessed June 1, 2021.
29. Palepu A, Carr PL, Friedman RH, et al. Specialty choices, compensation, and career satisfaction of underrepresented minority faculty in academic medicine. Acad Med 2000;75(2):157–60.
30. Yu PT, Parsa PV, Hassanein O, et al. Minorities struggle to advance in academic medicine: A 12-y review of diversity at the highest levels of America's teaching institutions. J Surg Res 2013;182(2):212–8.
31. Morgan A, Shah K, Tran K, et al. Racial, Ethnic, and Gender Representation in Leadership Positions at National Cancer Institute-Designated Cancer Centers. JAMA Netw Open 2021;4(6):e211280.

Disparities in the Management of Peritoneal Surface Malignancies

Kathleen Marulanda, MD, MS[a],
Ugwuji N. Maduekwe, MD, MMSc, MPH[b],*

KEYWORDS

- Disparities • Peritoneal malignancy • Carcinomatosis • Peritoneal metastases
- Ovarian cancer • Colorectal cancer • Appendiceal cancer • Cytoreductive surgery

KEY POINTS

- Cytoreductive surgery and hyperthermic intraperitoneal chemotherapy are recommended to optimize outcomes in select eligible patients with peritoneal metastases.
- Patients who are Black and/or with lower socioeconomic status are exposed to barriers of care that lead to decreased adherence to guideline-recommended therapies and worse survival.
- Racial disparities in survival for ovarian cancer are eliminated when patients receive National Comprehensive Cancer Network guideline-recommended treatment.

INTRODUCTION

Peritoneal metastases are a poor prognostic finding in a host of malignancies, including appendiceal neoplasms, gastric cancer, colorectal cancer, ovarian cancer, peritoneal mesothelioma, and primary peritoneal diseases. These aggressive malignancies are historically challenging to treat and associated with high morbidity and mortality. Consideration of the use of cytoreductive surgery (CRS) and hyperthermic intraperitoneal chemotherapy (HIPEC) to improve outcomes and survival is part of the modern approach to peritoneal involvement in these disease processes.[1–4] Cytoreduction involves complete resection of all macroscopic disease, often requiring extensive surgical resection, including complex peritonectomy, omentectomy, and multiple visceral resections for adequate control of tumor burden.[5] HIPEC following

[a] Department of Surgery, University of North Carolina, 4001 Burnett-Womack Building 170 Manning Drive, CB #7050, Chapel Hill, NC 27599-7050, USA; [b] Division of Surgical Oncology and Endocrine Surgery, Department of Surgery, University of North Carolina, 170 Manning Drive, CB #7213, Chapel Hill, NC 27599-7213, USA
* Corresponding author.
E-mail address: umaduekwe@mcw.edu
Twitter: kmaruMD (K.M.); umaduekwemd (U.N.M.)

Surg Oncol Clin N Am 31 (2022) 29–41
https://doi.org/10.1016/j.soc.2021.07.005
1055-3207/22/© 2021 Elsevier Inc. All rights reserved.

cytoreduction helps eradicate any residual microscopic disease in the peritoneal cavity. Recent data demonstrate superior outcomes and improved survival in select patients with ovarian, gastrointestinal, and appendiceal malignancies that are treated with CRS-HIPEC.[6–14]

Despite a growing body of evidence supporting its use,[15–18] widespread implementation of CRS-HIPEC remains a significant challenge. CRS-HIPEC is a resource-intensive proposition. Furthermore, differences in geographic and institutional distribution of expertise introduce variations in access and may leave vulnerable populations without this treatment option. In this review, we examine the current evidence regarding disparities in the management of peritoneal surface malignancies and aim to identify the predominant factors that drive disparities in care.

DISPARITIES IN PERITONEAL SURFACE MALIGNANCIES

Racial/ethnic disparities in the management of peritoneal surface malignancies lead to worse outcomes and increased mortality. Disparities may be related to multiple factors, including (1) cancer stage at diagnosis, (2) tumor biology, (3) response to and efficacy of treatment, (4) receipt of optimal treatment options, and/or (5) varying combinations of the aforementioned factors.

A broad spectrum of disease is included under the umbrella term "peritoneal surface malignancies." Here, we focus on peritoneal disease arising from ovarian, appendiceal, and colorectal sources, as these variants have the greatest breadth of data with CRS and intraperitoneal chemotherapy.

OVARIAN CANCER

One of the first diseases for which management incorporated the principles of CRS[19] and/or intraperitoneal chemotherapy,[13,20] ovarian cancer has the most disparities-related literature among anatomic sources of peritoneal surface malignancy, with extensive evidence linking race to survival.[21,22] Despite therapeutic advances and overall improvement in survival trends, racial disparities in all-cause mortality have worsened over time.[23] Despite experiencing lower incidence of ovarian cancer,[24,25] Black women have 1.3 times higher risk of all-cause mortality compared with White women.[23] A population-based study with Surveillance, Epidemiology, and End Results (SEER) data from 1988 to 1997 found that Black women had nearly 1 year shorter median crude survival compared with White women (22 vs 32 months).[24] More recently, national data from 1975 to 2016 showed that the 5-year survival rate in White women increased from 33% to 48%, while dropping from 44% to 41% in Black women.[26]

Stage at Presentation

Ovarian cancer survival is directly related to stage at the time of diagnosis: 5-year overall survival (OS) is 11% for stage IV disease compared with 88% for stage I disease.[24] Disparities may be related to Black women being more likely to present with advanced stages of disease[21,22,27,28]; a SEER data analysis found that 41% of Black women presented with stage IV disease compared with 34% of White women ($P < .0001$).[21] However, this stage distribution difference does not wholly account for survival differences. A case-control study across 47 hospitals in Cook County, Illinois, demonstrated worse survival in Black patients compared with White patients despite no significant difference in rates of advanced stage at diagnosis (52.9% vs 51.7%, respectively).[29] Even after adjusting for potential confounders, Black women remained 2.2 times more likely to die from ovarian cancer compared with White women.

Tumor Biology

Certain genetic mutations have been associated with increased ovarian cancer risk in specific racial groups.[30,31] For example, a short peptide (CAG) expressed on androgen receptors was associated with a twofold increased risk of ovarian cancer in Black patients with no similar effect in White patients.[31] Molecular composition may also alter treatment efficacy. A retrospective single-institution analysis of 393 patients showed that Black women had more than twice the rate of platinum resistance compared with White women (35% vs 14%), and, after adjusting for socioeconomic status (SES) and treatment factors, they were also found to have a survival disadvantage, as evidenced by lower progression-free survival (16 vs 27 months, $P = .003$) and OS (42 vs 88 months, $P < .001$).[32] Other multi-institutional and population-based studies, however, have not shown racial differences in tumor histology and/or grade.[24,29,33] Interestingly, a racial gap in outcomes only developed in the 1980s after CRS in combination with platinum-based chemotherapy was adopted as the treatment of choice for advanced disease. Before this, unadjusted survival rates were comparable between racial cohorts,[34] suggesting that survival advantages are more likely associated with access to care than with biologic differences.

Therapeutic Response and Efficacy

Treatment-related mortality

Aggressive treatment with CRS is not without risk. Primary cytoreduction for gynecologic malignancies is associated with 22% major morbidity and 1.4% mortality within 30 days of surgery.[35] However, risk may not be evenly distributed across racial groups. A SEER population-based cohort study evaluating perioperative mortality in common cancers found that non-White patients with ovarian cancer were more likely to die within 1 month after cancer-directed surgery than White patients (adjusted odds ratio [OR] 1.23; 95% confidence interval [CI] 1.08–1.39, $P = .002$).[36] In another SEER study examining perioperative mortality after primary CRS, patients admitted emergently had a threefold higher risk of dying within 30 days after surgery compared with those who were admitted electively (20.12% vs 5.56%, $P < .001$) and emergent admissions were more likely in non-White patients ($P < .001$).[37] Although race was not directly correlated with perioperative mortality, it did serve as an indirect marker of risk of exposure to worse outcomes given its association with emergent admissions.[37]

Treatment efficacy

Many studies demonstrate that when Black and White patients receive the same care, stage-specific survival is equivalent.[33,38,39] A population-based study of 4262 patients with ovarian cancer found a 50% risk reduction in all-cause mortality following cancer-directed surgery and adjuvant chemotherapy.[40] The improved survival benefit was comparable in both Black and White women when adjusted for treatment (hazard ratio [HR] 0.93; 95% CI 0.82–1.06). In a different SEER-based study, Cox regression analysis adjusted for patient and tumor characteristics found higher mortality rates in Black women (adjusted HR 1.17; 95% CI 1.02–1.35).[22] Yet, when treatment was accounted for, propensity-matched cohorts no longer showed any racial differences in OS rates (adjusted HR 1.06; 95% CI 0.84–1.34), indicating that racial disparities may be explained by differences in care. In additional support of this theory, a review of 1392 women enrolled in multiple clinical trials and treated with National

Comprehensive Cancer Network (NCCN)-recommended platinum-based chemotherapy demonstrated no difference in progression-free survival or OS across racial groups.[41]

Single-institution studies provide more discrete information about the specifics of treatment and patient demographics. A study of 209 women treated at a large academic center demonstrated similar survival rates across racial cohorts.[42] Race was not associated with survival after adjusting for multiple clinicodemographic factors, including sensitivity to chemotherapy and completion of cytoreduction. Of note, nearly all Black patients in this study were insured versus the national average of only 50%, a factor that may, in part, explain these outcomes. The investigators also did not differentiate between different treatment modalities, that is, extent of CRS or dose/routing of specific chemotherapy regimens. In a similar study, 405 patients treated at a tertiary referral center demonstrated no racial differences in survival on multivariate analysis.[33] In the latter study, Black and White women had near-identical rates of optimal cytoreduction (69% vs 73%, $P = .28$), complete removal of gross disease (54% vs 51%, $P = .49$), platinum-based and taxane-based chemotherapy (87% vs 88%, $P = .55$), intraperitoneal chemotherapy (18% vs 17%, $P = .56$), and 6 or more cycles of chemotherapy (85% vs 84%, $P = .72$).

Receipt of Therapy

Unfortunately, only 44% of patients with ovarian cancer receive NCCN guideline-adherent care,[43] despite guideline adherence having been shown to be an independent predictor of increased disease-specific survival.[44] In nationally representative data, significant differences in median disease-specific survival were reported between patients who received adherent care (36 months; 95% CI 35–38 months) versus those who did not (9 months; 95% CI 9–10 months, $P < .0001$),[44] and nonadherence was associated with a 60% increase in disease-specific mortality in propensity-matched cohorts.[44] Multivariate logistic regression analysis identified Black race as an independent predictor of guideline nonadherence (adjusted OR 1.53; 95% CI 1.22–1.92),[44] with the increased likelihood of receiving substandard care as a mediator of the relationship between Black race and worse outcomes. Improved adherence resulted in near-identical and reproducible survival benefits in all race/ethnicity and socioeconomic cohorts. This finding is likely because receipt of adherent treatment has been associated with a higher likelihood of receiving optimal cytoreduction (77.8% vs 54.4%, $P < .001$).[45] More stringent adherence to standardized care can benefit all patients and may help eliminate outcome disparities.

Failure to receive recommended cytoreductive surgery

A SEER database study found that Black women had a 40% increased risk of not receiving surgery compared with White women.[24] Multivariate analysis in another population-based study showed a higher likelihood of receiving surgery among White compared with Black patients (OR 1.41; 95% CI 1.10–1.82, $P = .007$).[46] Among 2766 patients from the Illinois State Cancer Registry, Black women were less likely to undergo debulking surgery (OR 0.39; 95% CI 0.30–0.50) or any surgery (OR 0.38; 95% CI 0.29–0.49) after adjusting for relevant covariates.[47] Similarly, a meta-analysis showed a decreased likelihood of having any type surgery among Black women compared with White women (pooled relative risk [RR] 1.17; 95% CI 1.10–1.23).[38] Lower rates of cancer-directed surgery have been used to explain worse survival in Black patients,[33,38,48] as evidence has shown that failure to undergo surgery is associated with an HR of 2.6 for all-cause mortality.[24]

Failure to receive recommended chemotherapy
Data from a statewide cancer registry found that after controlling for relevant factors, Black women were less likely to receive multi-agent chemotherapy (OR 0.56; 95% CI 0.45–0.71) or any type of chemotherapy (OR 0.58; 95% CI 0.45–0.74) compared with White women.[47] A propensity score matching analysis of SEER data found that Black women were less likely to receive complete treatment regimens compared with White women (54% vs 66%, $P < .03$).[22] Specifically, Black women had lower receipt of adjuvant chemotherapy despite having similar rates of surgery.[22] Decreased administration of chemotherapy in Black women persisted even when controlling for SES (50.2% vs 64.7%, $P < .001$).[40] Based on nationally representative data, Black women are 20% less likely than White women to be treated in accordance with NCCN guidelines.[49]

Factors related to underutilization of recommended therapy
Black patients have been shown to be less likely to be treated by a high-volume surgeon,[48] and women who receive care from high-volume, specialized surgeons are more likely to receive guideline-adherent care.[50,51] Care from specialized physicians may result in better OS,[51] although this association has not been consistently demonstrated in the literature.[52] Hospital characteristics, including type (teaching vs nonteaching) and volume (high vs low) have also been implicated, with lower volume being associated with a higher likelihood of receiving substandard care.[50] Location may also affect outcomes. A study found that patients treated in the Northeast region of the United States and those who lived near their treating hospital were more likely to receive chemotherapy as their primary treatment.[53] Because primary chemotherapy is typically designated for more severe disease and often considered a suboptimal option, these findings suggest that physician expertise and institutional familiarity with the disease may dictate the treatment options that patients are offered. Notably, a retrospective study from a high-volume NCCN cancer center calls into question the importance of high-volume surgeons and hospitals, as it demonstrated that even in this setting, not all patients had equal receipt of comprehensive guideline-adherent care.[45] This study suggested that patient factors related to adherence were the most common reason for not receiving NCCN-adhered care, specifically, failure to complete chemotherapy, which was most often ascribed to patient comorbidities and progression of disease.[45] The complex, intricate relationship among physician, hospital, and patient factors cannot be overlooked when investigating the mechanisms behind decreased utilization of standardized care.

APPENDICEAL CANCER

Appendiceal cancer is a rare disease affecting 0.12 per 100,000 people per year in the United States with 5-year OS rates as low as 38%.[54] Holowatyj and colleagues[55] was the first to study the impact of race/ethnicity on survival in young patients with appendiceal cancer in the United States in 2020. A total of 1652 patients from the SEER data registry were analyzed and results showed a significant difference in 5-year OS among White, Black, and Hispanic patients (75.5% vs 63% vs 75.4%, $P = .001$). After adjustment, Cox proportional hazard analysis found higher overall (HR 1.47; 95% CI 1.10–1.95) and cancer-specific (HR 1.47; 95% CI 1.10–1.98) mortality in Black versus White patients. Multivariate analysis in another SEER-based study also identified race as independently associated with outcomes.[56] These findings suggest that race may be associated with outcomes in appendiceal cancer.

Tumor Biology

Histologic tumor subtype was shown to be prognostic of racial disparities in survival in a large population-based study.[55] Among young patients with mucinous histology, Black patients had lower overall (HR 1.96; 95% CI 1.27–3.04) and disease-specific survival (HR 2.04; 95% CI 1.30–3.18) compared with White patients.[55] Another SEER database study found that race was significantly associated with differences in distribution of tumor histology (P < .001).[56] The most aggressive subtype, signet ring cell, was most commonly found in Asian/Pacific Islander patients.

Receipt of Therapy

Poor guideline adoption is common in appendiceal cancer. A population-based study of 18,055 patients from the National Cancer Database (NCDB) (2004–2014) found that only 7.7% of patients received CRS and perioperative intraperitoneal chemotherapy.[57] White race (OR 2.0; 95% CI 1.40–2.86) and non-Hispanic ethnicity (OR 1.92; 95% CI 1.21–3.05) were both predictors of increased likelihood of undergoing CRS-HIPEC, and receipt was associated with higher 5-year OS compared with surgery alone (65.6% vs 62.4%, P < .01). Another study using the NCDB registry identified 1190 patients who underwent CRS-HIPEC and found no difference in survival based on race.[58]

Factors related to underutilization of recommended therapy

Geographic location. In a nationally representative study using NCDB data, patients in the South Atlantic region of the United States were more likely to receive CRS and intraperitoneal chemotherapy compared with other areas of the country (OR 2.40; 95% CI 1.96–2.93).[57] Notably, patients undergoing CRS and intraperitoneal chemotherapy were more likely to travel longer distances to receive care, and every additional 25 miles traveled was associated with a 3% increase in likelihood of receiving CRS and perioperative intraperitoneal chemotherapy (1.03; 95% CI 1.02–1.04).[57]

Access to care. Although insurance status does not necessarily translate into access to care, it is an important and often critical factor for access to treatment, particularly in the United States. An NCDB data analysis showed that patients with private insurance were more likely to receive appropriate CRS-HIPEC (OR 1.52; 95% CI 1.26–1.84).[57] Receipt of NCCN-adherent therapy translated into higher 5-year survival compared with receipt of surgery alone (P < .01). This finding suggests that insurance status may serve as a surrogate of NCCN adherence, and therefore, may be indirectly associated with better outcomes.

COLORECTAL CANCER
Receipt of Therapy

Factors related to underutilization of recommended therapy

Socioeconomic status. In 2015, Tabrizian and colleagues[59] evaluated 448 patients who sought surgical treatment for colorectal cancer at their institution: 224 underwent colectomy for nonmetastatic disease, 112 hepatectomy for liver metastases, and 112 CRS-HIPEC for peritoneal metastases. They found that most patients treated with CRS-HIPEC were White, English-speaking, had private insurance, and traveled greater distances to receive care.[59] Multivariate analysis demonstrated that, compared with other surgical options, receipt of CRS-HIPEC was associated with younger age, farther traveling distance, and private insurance. Another recent large cohort study from a single high-volume center found that low SES was an independent predictor of worse perioperative outcomes and OS.[60] Compared with patients from higher socioeconomic backgrounds, those with low SES had longer lengths of stay (12 vs 11 days, $P = .01$), more complications (inpatient comprehensive complication index score 23 vs 21, $P = .01$), and higher 90-day readmission (51% vs 33%, $P = .01$) and 30-day mortality rates (5% vs 0%, $P = .02$). The low-SES cohort was less likely to receive adjuvant chemotherapy after CRS-HIPEC (43% vs 60%, $P = .02$), and median OS was significantly worse for them versus the high-SES cohort following CRS-HIPEC (17.8 vs 32.4 months, $P = .02$). Interestingly, the high-SES group tended to have more aggressive tumor phenotypes, so tumor biology was likely not the cause of these disparities, although it is possible that tumor biology was a mediator and led to higher referral rates in the high-SES cohort. Although both groups had similar time to progression, the low-SES cohort had worse survival rates, suggesting that differences in survival may be driven by variations in long-term management. Both adjuvant chemotherapy and repeat CRS-HIPEC were less common in the low-SES group and, on multivariate analysis, SES was an independent predictor for increased mortality, even when controlling for receipt of adjuvant chemotherapy and repeat CRS-HIPEC.

Physician knowledge and expertise. Referral patterns to HIPEC centers remain largely predicated on physician preference. A multistate study surveyed physicians who care for patients with gastrointestinal cancer and found notable discrepancies in knowledge about and utilization of HIPEC.[61] More than 50% of respondents underestimated 5-year survival following CRS-HIPEC while simultaneously overestimating the procedure's perioperative mortality. Inadequate access to an HIPEC specialist and misconceptions regarding treatment efficacy were the most common reasons cited for not referring patients to an HIPEC center. This finding reflects the potential for implicit bias in referral, as physicians may be less likely to refer patients from low socioeconomic backgrounds for more advanced procedures. This tendency has been previously reported for other procedures, including cardiac catherization,[59] and is rooted in the assumption that low-SES groups are less likely to comply and follow up with care. As a result, these patients are offered fewer options and receive substandard care.

RECOMMENDATIONS AND FUTURE DIRECTIONS

The existence of sociodemographic disparities in the surgical management of peritoneal surface malignancies is largely undisputed, but its driving mechanisms are still debated. Current data suggest that barriers in access to high-volume/high-performing peritoneal surface malignancy centers disproportionately affect Black and Hispanic patients, those with lower SES, those insured with Medicare, and those with more comorbidities. In ovarian cancer, in particular, SES appears to be the strongest predictor of decreased survival, presumably because SES serves as a proxy for decreased access and increased likelihood of receiving nonadherent therapy.

Approaching disparities through a lens in which distinctions are made between race and other social determinants of health is not unreasonable, but such an approach is predicated on the belief that a patient's genetic composition is not directly and tightly intertwined with environmental and societal pressures, and, therefore, somewhat limits our interpretation and analysis of disparities research. To better understand the relationship between race and cancer outcomes, the Ecosocial Theory of Disease Distribution and its concept of embodiment must be considered.[62] Embodiment describes how the human body is the physical and biological manifestation of societal and ecological forces. Thus, differences in distribution of diseases are an embodiment of how varying physiologic, behavioral, and genetic exposures can impact the human body at the molecular level. Another important lens through which to contextualize the framework in which we interpret racialized outcomes is Fundamental Cause Theory, which acknowledges the persistent relationship between SES and overall mortality.[63,64] It highlights how patient outcomes and the curability of specific diseases continually depend on a patient's SES in society, and by extension, their accessibility to resources to help them combat disease. These concepts are necessary to adequately appreciate how racism, which is deeply interwoven into our society and manifested in profound socioeconomic inequity and significant physiologic stressors that directly impact the human experience, has a causative effect on patient outcomes and worsening disparities. A review study by Doll[65] was the first to investigate the role of racism on disparities in gynecologic cancers and emphasized the importance of using the proper framework to analyze results to properly interpret how racism impacts distribution of care.

To improve outcomes, we must recognize and address the dynamic ways structural factors influence our health care system's ability to successfully provide equal care to all patient populations. Systemic efforts to fund research that focuses on closing the gap in understanding between providers and the patient's experience can help mitigate factors that influence patient health. Greater emphasis on recruiting patients from different racial, geographic, and financial backgrounds can make research results more applicable to our entire patient population rather than a select few. National databases and clinical trials must incorporate data on patient sociodemographic characteristics beyond race and ethnicity to identify the variables that impact outcomes, quality of life, and overall health status. Furthermore, involvement of patients from diverse backgrounds in research studies will allow them to vocalize their concerns and their stressors during the investigative period, thus providing invaluable information regarding factors that drive disparities. This opportunity may also empower patients from marginalized communities to garner the knowledge they need to become their own advocates, an invaluable tool for ensuring that patients receive adequate care. Greater awareness of health care disparities among medical providers and more general understanding of malignant disease processes, specifically regarding the use of CRS-HIPEC to treat various peritoneal malignancies, may help to minimize physician bias.

Growing evidence shows that when patients receive standardized care, the racial gap disappears and comparable stage-specific outcomes are achieved. Adherence to guideline-recommended therapies should be prioritized to help mitigate disparities in peritoneal surface malignancies. The challenge then becomes how to provide guideline-adherent therapy to all patients. Support for centralized care is founded on the principle that high-volume physicians are more likely to comply with NCCN guidelines and provide comprehensive care resulting in improved outcomes. Cost analysis regarding centralization of care for advanced ovarian cancer found greater quality-adjusted life years due to higher rates of optimal debulking in high-volume centers.[66] Although these results are promising, centralized care also introduces temporal and economic burdens that affect feasibility and present additional barriers to access. Establishing a centralized care system in the United States may also pose its own set of challenges. It is unclear whether current high-volume centers can support an acute increase in patient load if all cases are reallocated to these few NCCN centers. The additional volume may overwhelm the existing system and create shortages. Thus, a balance must be struck between quality care, patient comfort, and feasibility, but ultimately, it is our responsibility as medical providers to ensure that all treatment options are presented to all patients.

CLINICS CARE POINTS

- Black women with ovarian cancer have 1.3 times higher risk of all-cause mortality after adjusting for age, tumor stage, marital status, and time of diagnosis. Propensity-matched cohorts adjusted for treatment do not exhibit racial differences in survival between Black and White patients with ovarian cancer (adjusted HR 1.06; 95% CI 0.84–1.34).[23]

- Black women with ovarian cancer are 20% less likely to receive NCCN guideline-recommended therapy, but racial differences in care receipt disappear after adjusting for age, marital status, comorbidity index, insurance status, and hospital characteristics.[49]

- In patients with colorectal peritoneal metastases, low SES is a significant predictor for not receiving debulking surgery or surgery without chemotherapy (OR 1.67; 95% CI 1.38–2.03), having an increased likelihood of receiving no treatment at all (OR 1.95; 95% CI 1.44–2.64), and significantly worse median OS following CRS-HIPEC compared with having high SES (17.8 vs 32.4 months, $P = .02$).[60]

- High-volume physicians managing ovarian cancer have higher debulking rates and are 5 times more likely to properly stage patients compared with those who provide care in low-volume centers. Multivariate analysis of patients treated by high-volume specialists with near-identical rates of optimal cytoreduction, complete resection of gross disease, and use of intraperitoneal and intravenous chemotherapy demonstrated similar survival and perioperative outcomes across racial groups.[33]

DISCLOSURE

UNM was supported by the UNC Oncology Clinical Translational Research Training Program (K12CA120780).

REFERENCES

1. Shaib WL, Assi R, Shamseddine A, et al. Appendiceal mucinous neoplasms: diagnosis and management. Oncologist 2017;22(9):1107–16.
2. Rizvi SA, Syed W, Shergill R. Approach to pseudomyxoma peritonei. World J Gastrointest Surg 2018;10(5):49–56.
3. (NCCN) NCCN. Guidelines for ovarian cancer (version 1.2019, March 8, 2019). NCCN; 2019.
4. Klaver CE, Groenen H, Morton DG, et al. Recommendations and consensus on the treatment of peritoneal metastases of colorectal origin: a systematic review of national and international guidelines. Colorectal Dis 2017;19(3):224–36.
5. The Chicago Consensus on Peritoneal Surface Malignancies: management of appendiceal neoplasms. Ann Surg Oncol 2020;27(6):1753–60.
6. Verwaal VJ, Bruin S, Boot H, et al. 8-year follow-up of randomized trial: cytoreduction and hyperthermic intraperitoneal chemotherapy versus systemic chemotherapy in patients with peritoneal carcinomatosis of colorectal cancer. Ann Surg Oncol 2008;15(9):2426–32.
7. Verwaal VJ, van Ruth S, de Bree E, et al. Randomized trial of cytoreduction and hyperthermic intraperitoneal chemotherapy versus systemic chemotherapy and palliative surgery in patients with peritoneal carcinomatosis of colorectal cancer. J Clin Oncol 2003;21(20):3737–43.
8. Sugarbaker PH. New standard of care for appendiceal epithelial neoplasms and pseudomyxoma peritonei syndrome? Lancet Oncol 2006;7(1):69–76.

9. Ellis RJ, Schlick CJR, Yang AD, et al. Utilization and treatment patterns of cytoreduction surgery and intraperitoneal chemotherapy in the United States. Ann Surg Oncol 2020;27(1):214–21.

10. Guerrero W, Munene G, Dickson PV, et al. Outcome and factors associated with aborted cytoreduction for peritoneal carcinomatosis. J Gastrointest Oncol 2018; 9(4):664–73.

11. Alberts DS, Liu PY, Hannigan EV, et al. Intraperitoneal cisplatin plus intravenous cyclophosphamide versus intravenous cisplatin plus intravenous cyclophosphamide for stage III ovarian cancer. N Engl J Med 1996;335(26):1950–5.

12. Armstrong DK, Bundy B, Wenzel L, et al. Intraperitoneal cisplatin and paclitaxel in ovarian cancer. N Engl J Med 2006;354(1):34–43.

13. van Driel WJ, Koole SN, Sikorska K, et al. Hyperthermic intraperitoneal chemotherapy in ovarian cancer. N Engl J Med 2018;378(3):230–40.

14. McMullen JRW, Selleck M, Wall NR, et al. Peritoneal carcinomatosis: limits of diagnosis and the case for liquid biopsy. Oncotarget 2017;8(26):43481–90.

15. Spiliotis J, Halkia E, de Bree E. Treatment of peritoneal surface malignancies with hyperthermic intraperitoneal chemotherapy-current perspectives. Curr Oncol 2016;23(3):e266–75.

16. Witkamp AJ, de Bree E, Van Goethem R, et al. Rationale and techniques of intraoperative hyperthermic intraperitoneal chemotherapy. Cancer Treat Rev 2001; 27(6):365–74.

17. Franko J, Ibrahim Z, Gusani NJ, et al. Cytoreductive surgery and hyperthermic intraperitoneal chemoperfusion versus systemic chemotherapy alone for colorectal peritoneal carcinomatosis. Cancer 2010;116(16):3756–62.

18. Sugarbaker PH. Peritoneal carcinomatosis: natural history and rational therapeutic interventions using intraperitoneal chemotherapy. Cancer Treat Res 1996;81: 149–68.

19. The Chicago Consensus on peritoneal surface malignancies: Standards. Cancer 2020;126(11):2516–24.

20. Riggs MJ, Pandalai PK, Kim J, et al. Hyperthermic intraperitoneal chemotherapy in ovarian cancer. Diagnostics (Basel) 2020;10(1):43.

21. Chan JK, Zhang M, Hu JM, et al. Racial disparities in surgical treatment and survival of epithelial ovarian cancer in United States. J Surg Oncol 2008;97(2):103–7.

22. Howell EA, Egorova N, Hayes MP, et al. Racial disparities in the treatment of advanced epithelial ovarian cancer. Obstet Gynecol 2013;122(5):1025–32.

23. Terplan M, Schluterman N, McNamara EJ, et al. Have racial disparities in ovarian cancer increased over time? An analysis of SEER data. Gynecol Oncol 2012; 125(1):19–24.

24. Barnholtz-Sloan JS, Tainsky MA, Abrams J, et al. Ethnic differences in survival among women with ovarian carcinoma. Cancer 2002;94(6):1886–93.

25. Ries LAGKC, Hankey BF, Miller BA, et al, editors. SEER cancer Statistics review, 1973-1994. Bethesda: National Cancer Institute. NIH; 1997. Pub. No. 97-2789.

26. Ovarian Cancer Studies Aim to Reduce Racial Disparities, Improve Outcomes. National Cancer Institute; 2020. Available at: https://www.cancer.gov/news-events/cancer-currents-blog/2020/ovarian-cancer-racial-disparities-studies.

27. Miller EM, Tymon-Rosario J, Strickler HD, et al. Racial differences in survival from epithelial ovarian cancer are associated with stage at diagnosis and use of neoadjuvant therapy: a 10-year single-institution experience with a racially diverse urban population. Int J Gynecol Cancer 2018;28(4):749–56.

28. Parham G, Phillips JL, Hicks ML, et al. The National Cancer Data Base report on malignant epithelial ovarian carcinoma in African-American women. Cancer 1997;80(4):816–26.
29. Kim S, Dolecek TA, Davis FG. Racial differences in stage at diagnosis and survival from epithelial ovarian cancer: a fundamental cause of disease approach. Soc Sci Med 2010;71(2):274–81.
30. Schildkraut JM, Goode EL, Clyde MA, et al. Single nucleotide polymorphisms in the TP53 region and susceptibility to invasive epithelial ovarian cancer. Cancer Res 2009;69(6):2349–57.
31. Schildkraut JM, Murphy SK, Palmieri RT, et al. Trinucleotide repeat polymorphisms in the androgen receptor gene and risk of ovarian cancer. Cancer Epidemiol Biomarkers Prev 2007;16(3):473–80.
32. Ross J, Braswell KV, Madeira da Silva L, et al. Unraveling the etiology of ovarian cancer racial disparity in the deep south: Is it nature or nurture? Gynecol Oncol 2017;145(2):329–33.
33. Bristow RE, Ueda S, Gerardi MA, et al. Analysis of racial disparities in stage IIIC epithelial ovarian cancer care and outcomes in a tertiary gynecologic oncology referral center. Gynecol Oncol 2011;122(2):319–23.
34. Barnholtz-Sloan JS, Schwartz AG, Qureshi F, et al. Ovarian cancer: changes in patterns at diagnosis and relative survival over the last three decades. Am J Obstet Gynecol 2003;189(4):1120–7.
35. Chi DS, Zivanovic O, Levinson KL, et al. The incidence of major complications after the performance of extensive upper abdominal surgical procedures during primary cytoreduction of advanced ovarian, tubal, and peritoneal carcinomas. Gynecol Oncol 2010;119(1):38–42.
36. Mahal BA, Inverso G, Aizer AA, et al. Incidence and determinants of 1-month mortality after cancer-directed surgery. Ann Oncol 2015;26(2):399–406.
37. Thrall MM, Goff BA, Symons RG, et al. Thirty-day mortality after primary cytoreductive surgery for advanced ovarian cancer in the elderly. Obstet Gynecol 2011;118(3):537–47.
38. Terplan M, Smith EJ, Temkin SM. Race in ovarian cancer treatment and survival: a systematic review with meta-analysis. Cancer Causes Control 2009;20(7):1139–50.
39. Brawley OW, Freeman HP. Race and outcomes: is this the end of the beginning for minority health research? J Natl Cancer Inst 1999;91(22):1908–9.
40. Du XL, Sun CC, Milam MR, et al. Ethnic differences in socioeconomic status, diagnosis, treatment, and survival among older women with epithelial ovarian cancer. Int J Gynecol Cancer 2008;18(4):660–9.
41. Farley JH, Tian C, Rose GS, et al. Race does not impact outcome for advanced ovarian cancer patients treated with cisplatin/paclitaxel: an analysis of Gynecologic Oncology Group trials. Cancer 2009;115(18):4210–7.
42. Terplan M, Temkin S, Tergas A, et al. Does equal treatment yield equal outcomes? The impact of race on survival in epithelial ovarian cancer. Gynecol Oncol 2008;111(2):173–8.
43. Thrall MM, Gray HJ, Symons RG, et al. Trends in treatment of advanced epithelial ovarian cancer in the Medicare population. Gynecol Oncol 2011;122(1):100–6.
44. Bristow RE, Chang J, Ziogas A, et al. Sociodemographic disparities in advanced ovarian cancer survival and adherence to treatment guidelines. Obstet Gynecol 2015;125(4):833–42.
45. Erickson BK, Martin JY, Shah MM, et al. Reasons for failure to deliver National Comprehensive Cancer Network (NCCN)-adherent care in the treatment of

epithelial ovarian cancer at an NCCN cancer center. Gynecol Oncol 2014;133(2): 142–6.

46. Fairfield KM, Lucas FL, Earle CC, et al. Regional variation in cancer-directed surgery and mortality among women with epithelial ovarian cancer in the Medicare population. Cancer 2010;116(20):4840–8.

47. Joslin CE, Brewer KC, Davis FG, et al. The effect of neighborhood-level socioeconomic status on racial differences in ovarian cancer treatment in a population-based analysis in Chicago. Gynecol Oncol 2014;135(2):285–91.

48. Bristow RE, Zahurak ML, Ibeanu OA. Racial disparities in ovarian cancer surgical care: a population-based analysis. Gynecol Oncol 2011;121(2):364–8.

49. Harlan LC, Clegg LX, Trimble EL. Trends in surgery and chemotherapy for women diagnosed with ovarian cancer in the United States. J Clin Oncol 2003;21(18): 3488–94.

50. Goff BA, Matthews BJ, Larson EH, et al. Predictors of comprehensive surgical treatment in patients with ovarian cancer. Cancer 2007;109(10):2031–42.

51. Earle CC, Schrag D, Neville BA, et al. Effect of surgeon specialty on processes of care and outcomes for ovarian cancer patients. J Natl Cancer Inst 2006;98(3): 172–80.

52. Schrag D, Earle C, Xu F, et al. Associations between hospital and surgeon procedure volumes and patient outcomes after ovarian cancer resection. J Natl Cancer Inst 2006;98(3):163–71.

53. Hinchcliff E, Melamed A, Bregar A, et al. Factors associated with delivery of neoadjuvant chemotherapy in women with advanced stage ovarian cancer. Gynecol Oncol 2018;148(1):168–73.

54. Marmor S, Portschy PR, Tuttle TM, et al. The Rise in appendiceal cancer incidence: 2000-2009. J Gastrointest Surg 2015;19(4):743–50.

55. Holowatyj AN, Washington KM, Salaria SN, et al. Early-onset appendiceal cancer survival by race or ethnicity in the United States. Gastroenterology 2020;159(4): 1605–8.

56. Mo S, Zhou Z, Ying Z, et al. Epidemiology of and prognostic factors for appendiceal carcinomas: a retrospective, population-based study. Int J Colorectal Dis 2019;34(11):1915–24.

57. Byrne RM, Gilbert EW, Dewey EN, et al. Who undergoes cytoreductive surgery and perioperative intraperitoneal chemotherapy for appendiceal cancer? An analysis of the National Cancer Database. J Surg Res 2019;238:198–206.

58. Rozich NS, Lewis SE, Chen S, et al. Women survive longer than men undergoing cytoreductive surgery and HIPEC for appendiceal cancer. PLoS One 2021;16(4): e0250726.

59. Tabrizian P, Overbey J, Carrasco-Avino G, et al. Escalation of socioeconomic disparities among patients with colorectal cancer receiving advanced surgical treatment. Ann Surg Oncol 2015;22(5):1746–50.

60. Rieser CJ, Hoehn RS, Zenati M, et al. Impact of Socioeconomic Status on Presentation and Outcomes in Colorectal Peritoneal Metastases Following Cytoreduction and Chemoperfusion: Persistent Inequalities in Outcomes at a High-Volume Center. Ann Surg Oncol 2021 Jul;28(7):3522–31.

61. Bernaiche T, Emery E, Bijelic L. Practice patterns, attitudes, and knowledge among physicians regarding cytoreductive surgery and HIPEC for patients with peritoneal metastases. Pleura Peritoneum 2018;3(1):20170025.

62. Krieger N. Theories for social epidemiology in the 21st century: an ecosocial perspective. Int J Epidemiol 2001;30(4):668–77.

63. Bor J, Cohen GH, Galea S. Population health in an era of rising income inequality: USA, 1980–2015. Lancet 2017;389(10077):1475–90.
64. Bailey ZD, Krieger N, Agénor M, et al. Structural racism and health inequities in the USA: evidence and interventions. Lancet 2017;389(10077):1453–63.
65. Doll KM. Investigating Black-White disparities in gynecologic oncology: Theories, conceptual models, and applications. Gynecol Oncol 2018;149(1):78–83.
66. Bristow RE, Santillan A, Diaz-Montes TP, et al. Centralization of care for patients with advanced-stage ovarian cancer: a cost-effectiveness analysis. Cancer 2007; 109(8):1513–22.

Undertreatment of Pancreatic Cancer
The Intersection of Bias, Biology, and Geography

Madeline B. Torres, MD[a], Matthew E.B. Dixon, MD[b],
Niraj J. Gusani, MD, MS[c],*

KEYWORDS

- Pancreatic cancer • Disparities • Race • Socioeconomic • Multimodality therapy
- Surgery • High volume

KEY POINTS

- Racial and socioeconomic disparities exist in the incidence and treatment of pancreatic cancer.
- Black, indigenous, and people of color (BIPOC) and socioeconomically disadvantaged patients receive less multimodality treatment and care at high-volume centers.
- BIPOC and elderly patients are underrepresented in clinical trials, raising concerns over the application of current recommendations to the general population.

INTRODUCTION

Pancreatic cancer (PC) is the third leading cause of cancer death in the United States.[1] PC is expected to surpass colorectal cancer to become the second leading cause of cancer death by 2030.[2] Despite advances in medicine and the increased utilization of immunotherapy, the overall survival of patients with PC remains poor, with a 10% survival rate at 5 years.[1,3]

[a] General Surgery, Department of Surgery, Penn State Health Milton S. Hershey Medical Center, 500 University Avenue MC H149, Hershey, PA 17033, USA; [b] Division of Surgical Oncology, Penn State Health Milton S. Hershey Medical Center, 500 University Avenue MC H070, Hershey, PA 17036, USA; [c] Section of Surgical Oncology, Baptist MD Anderson Cancer Center, 1301 Palm Avenue, Jacksonville, FL 32207, USA
* Corresponding author.
E-mail address: Niraj.Gusani@bmcjax.com
Twitter: @MadelineBTorres (M.B.T.); @mebdixon (M.E.B.D.); @NirajGusani (N.J.G.)

Surg Oncol Clin N Am 31 (2022) 43–54
https://doi.org/10.1016/j.soc.2021.07.006
1055-3207/22/© 2021 Elsevier Inc. All rights reserved.

It is well established that the incidence of PC, opportunities for treatment, and outcomes following therapy are dependent on tumor biology[4–8]; however, these entities are also influenced by an individual's race, gender, ethnicity, and socioeconomic staus.[1,9] Exposure to cancer risk factors as well as lack of access to basic preventive care, screening, and multimodality treatment at high-volume centers (HVCs) are largely determined by an individual's socioeconomic status (SES), education, employment, income, and insurance benefits, among other factors. Inequities in these factors disproportionately affect Black, indigenous, and people of color (BIPOC) patients and are exacerbated by this country's history of structural racism.[9,10] For example, patients who lived in areas of redlining, a form of lending discrimination, were found to experience a twofold increase in breast cancer mortality.[11] Black patients are affected disproportionately by PC, with increased incidence rates compared with White patients, whereas lower incidence has been observed among individuals who are Hispanic, Asian/Pacific Islander, or Native American.[3,12] Black patients have a 16% increased risk of death across all cancers, and experience worse survival from PC.[13–15]

The purpose of this article was to review social determinant factors that contribute to the undertreatment of PC and to examine the effects these factors have on patient outcomes.

EPIDEMIOLOGIC DISPARITIES

PC disproportionately affects Black patients. Blacks have higher PC incidence rates than any other racial/ethnic group at 15.3 per 100,000 compared with individuals who are non-Hispanic White (NHW, 13.3 per 100,000), American Indian (10 per 100,000), Hispanic (11.6 per 100,000), or Asian/Pacific Islander (10 per 100,000).[3,12] The explanation for this disparity in incidence is unknown, and likely multifactorial, but appears to be related to a variety of factors, including differential rates of smoking, exposure to chemicals, alcohol use, periodontal disease, diabetes, poverty, and obesity.[16–20]

PC mortality rates also differ by race. Black individuals experience the highest reported death rates (13.3 per 100,000), compared with those who are NHW (11.1 per 100,000), American Indian (6.6 per 100,000), Hispanic (8.5 per 100,000), or Asian/Pacific Islander (7.6 per 100,00).[3,21] However, with more granular examination, it becomes clear that other racial and ethnic groups also experience mortality-related disparity after PC diagnosis. Native American individuals experience worse survival than NHWs, with a reported 1-year survival rate of 26.2% compared with 48.3% for NHW patients.[22] Furthermore, Native American patients die at a higher rate within the first month of diagnosis compared with NHW patients (25.8% vs 7.5%, $P = .004$).[22] Notably, however, and likely also contributing to differential mortality, Black patients present more frequently with locoregional and metastatic disease, leading to lower rates of surgical resection.[23,24]

DIFFERENCES IN BIOLOGY

Racial differences in gene expression as well as tumor inflammatory response, behavior, and microenvironment have been previously reported in various cancers.[4–6] Although their significance in contributing to disparities in PC is unclear, it is important to mention their existence and examine their potential contribution. The presence of the KRAS mutation in PC has been correlated with aggressive disease and worse survival.[7] Although similar rates of KRAS mutations at codon 12 between Black and White patients have been reported, Pernick and colleagues[8,25,26] found higher rates of glycine-to-valine point mutations in Black patients, a finding that is, hypothesized to lead to more aggressive disease and worse survival.

The somatostatin subtype receptor SSTR5 has been associated with regulation of pancreatic cell tumorigenesis, and 3 genotypes have been identified.[27] The SSTR5 P109S variant has been associated with increased risk of PC, whereas the CC (proline) genotype is associated with increased tumor aggression and higher risk of mortality.[27,28] The CC genotype occurs more frequently in Black compared with White and Hispanic individuals, potentially contributing to the increased incidence of PC in Black individuals.[27,29] Furthermore, a small study reported increased DNA methylation rates in Black newborns at gene-containing cancer pathways known to be associated with increased rates of pancreatic, prostate, and bladder cancer, and melanoma, representing another potential mechanism for differential incidence.[30]

In addition, Kaiso, a bimodal transcription factor that facilitates tumorigenesis via methylation-dependent silencing of tumor suppressor genes, has elevated expression in Black patients with PC, and is associated with higher rates of invasive, node-positive disease.[27,31] Last, KDM4/JMJD2A, a histone demethylator, has increased expression in Black patients with PC and is associated with decreased disease-free survival; this potential mechanism, however, has not been well studied in other racial groups.[27,32] All of the previously mentioned transcription factors, receptors, and mutations have been associated with increased risk of developing PC or worse overall outcomes. Although they may contribute to the increased incidence and lower survival seen in Black patients with PC, they are not solely responsible for the disparity in outcomes.

TREATMENT PATTERNS AND UNDERUTILIZATION OF MULTIMODALITY CARE
Underutilization of Multimodality Treatment

More than 50% of patients with PC present with metastatic disease, 30% present with borderline resectable and locally advanced disease, and only 20% present with resectable disease at initial diagnosis.[33,34] Multimodality treatment, including surgery, renders the best chance of long-term survival.[3] Multiple studies have focused on differential evaluation and receipt of surgery based on race, most suggesting fewer offers to and less receipt of surgery by BIPOC patients and concomitantly lower survival rates.[35–38] In 2010, Riall and colleagues[39] reported 29% of Black patients with potentially resectable disease did not receive surgical evaluation and were also less likely to undergo surgical resection. More recently, Moaven and colleagues[38] demonstrated that Black patients were offered surgery at lower rates compared with White patients (22.9% vs 27.5%, $P\leq.001$).

Another retrospective study found surgical resection was recommended and performed less often among Black patients compared with White patients.[40] Similarly, when surgery was recommended, Black patients underwent fewer resections (16.6% vs 12.7%).[41] A single-institution study at an HVC reported that individuals who were older, had more comorbidities, and were non-English speaking were less likely to undergo surgery.[42] A National Cancer Database (NCDB) study from 1995 to 2004 reported patients who were Black, had lower incomes, came from less educated backgrounds, and had nonprivate insurance were less likely to undergo surgery.[37] The investigators found 38.2% of patients with potentially resectable PC were not offered surgery, whereas 51.7% of patients with stage I disease did not receive surgery due to comorbidities, advanced age, or patient refusal.[37] In 2016, Shapiro and colleagues[43] found Black patients were less likely to undergo resection compared with White patients (odds ratio [OR] 0.76; 95% confidence interval [CI] 0.65–0.88; $P<.001$). Similarly, American Indian patients had lower odds of resection, and Hispanic patients also experienced lower resection rates compared with non-Hispanic patients (OR 0.72; 95% CI 0.60–0.85; P<.001).[43]

Despite strong evidence supporting multimodality treatment, many BIPOC patients are not offered consultation and do not receive multimodality care. Black patients experience lower rates of specialist consultation,[22,35,36,44] including consultation with a medical oncologist (adjusted OR [AOR] 0.74, P<.01), radiation oncologist (AOR 0.75, P<.01), and surgical oncologist (AOR 0.71, P<.01).[41] Black patients are also less likely to undergo chemotherapy (AOR 0.59, P<.01). Another study found that Black patients are 25% less likely to receive adjuvant chemotherapy and 30% less likely to receive adjuvant chemoradiation.[35,44] In New Mexico, Native American patients with PC were also found to be less likely to be offered chemotherapy compared with NHW patients (OR 2.41, P = .26).[22] In unresectable disease, patients with private insurance were more likely to receive systemic therapy compared with those without insurance (P<.01).[45]

Factors Contributing to Underutilization of Multimodality Therapy

Multiple factors contribute to low specialist consultation, surgical resection rates, and receipt of multimodality therapy in BIPOC patients.[35,37,38,43,45–47] Cheung and colleagues[48] found that patients with low SES and multiple comorbidities were less likely to receive surgery, radiation, and chemotherapy.

Sridhar and colleagues[46] found that patients with private insurance experienced increased receipt of perioperative therapy compared with those with Medicaid or Medicare, or those who were uninsured. A study of the Florida Cancer Data System found that median survival in patients with PC was inversely associated with poverty levels, and private insurance was associated with longer median survival.[48] Loehrer and colleagues[49] evaluated the effect of health insurance expansion on treatment of PC in Massachusetts after the 2006 health care reform, and found increased resection rates for PC compared with states that did not expand access to health insurance. However, Chang and colleagues[24] found that Black patients still received surgery at lower rates (25%) compared with NHW (30.7%) and Hispanic (39.5%) patients after controlling for insurance status, suggesting that lack of insurance is not the sole contributing factor to decreased rates of resection.

Implicit bias and nihilism on the part of physicians also play a significant role in diagnosis, specialist referral, and treatment options provided to BIPOC patients.[50] Manfredi and colleagues[51] found that Black patients received less cancer information, including names of and referral to cancer specialists. Furthermore, physicians may be less patient-centered, provide poor quality information, and offer different advice when meeting Black patients.[15,52] Shah and colleagues[40] found that in patients with comparable disease stage, surgeons were less likely to recommend surgery to Black patients. This omission is potentially fueled by erroneous beliefs on the part of surgeons regarding worse outcomes in Black patients, misperceptions of Black patients as less intelligent and undereducated, and stereotypes of Black patients having poor social support and increased risk of noncompliance.[40,53,54] Indeed, Bilimoria and colleagues[37] hypothesized that the decreased offers for resection were due to nihilistic historical attitudes of poor outcomes in patients who undergo pancreatectomy.

Patient preference and refusal of surgery play important roles in treatment receipt as well, and misconceptions about cancer surgery may drive patient refusal to undergo surgery.[55] These beliefs may be mitigated by practicing culturally competent, patient-centered care to provide evidence in support of treatment and to explore and address patients' treatment-related concerns and anxieties. Notably, Black patients are 3 times more likely than White patients to refuse PC surgery,[56] and this finding may not be entirely due to differential rates of surgical recommendation. A 2009 Surveillance, Epidemiology, and End Results database study found that Black patients were more likely to refuse surgery despite equal recommendations for surgical resection.[41] Similarly, Shah and colleagues[40] found Black patients were more likely to refuse surgery. Refusal of surgery was associated with older age, evaluation at a nonacademic/research program, having more comorbidities, and having nonprivate insurance.[57] Patient refusal of surgery has also been associated with refusal of other therapy modalities, including radiation.[40] Reasons for refusal of treatment include historical distrust of the health care system, concerns for surgical risk, and perceived diagnostic uncertainty.[42,58,59] However, to simply state that patient mistrust contributes to the disparity in receipt of treatment among BIPOC patients is to ignore years of mistreatment, abuse, and racism heavily embedded in the history of medicine. Therefore, shifting blame to patient mistrust rather than focusing on addressing the racism that has contributed to both patient mistrust and documented health inequities will only perpetuate health care disparities.

REGIONALIZATION AND SEQUESTRATION AT HIGH-VOLUME CENTERS

Multiple studies have demonstrated the benefits of HVCs performing pancreatic surgery, including decreased mortality and morbidity, shorter length of stay, and lower hospital costs.[60–65] Furthermore, national cancer guidelines recommend pancreatic resections be performed at HVCs.[19]

The effect of regionalization and sequestration at HVCs goes beyond improved outcomes and has been associated with increased receipt of multimodality therapy and increased rates of negative resection margins. A 2007 study of the NCDB by Bilimoria and colleagues[66] demonstrated that patients who received therapy at academic HVCs were more likely to receive multimodality therapy. Furthermore, a systematic review of the literature found that, among patients who underwent pancreaticoduodenectomy (ie, the Whipple procedure) for PC, there was an association between volume and negative margin rates,[67] 76% at very-HVCs versus 55% at LVCs ($P = .008$), and also reported higher 5-year survival rates at higher volume sites.[67]

Despite evidence supporting regionalization of care at HVCs, unequal referral to HVCs has been reported.[68] Evaluation of the patients undergoing surgical resection in the National Inpatient Sample (NIS) found that Asian/Pacific Islander and other non-White patients, those with nonprivate insurance, and those with multiple comorbidities were more likely to receive pancreatectomy at low-volume centers (LVCs) (57.3%).[69] These findings were further validated by Bliss and colleagues,[68] whose review of the NIS data from 2004 to 2011 reported more comorbidities ($P = .001$), lower rates of private insurance ($P<.001$), and more nonelective admissions in patients undergoing surgical resection at LVCs. Epstein and colleagues[70] reported Black patients were less likely to receive surgery by a high-volume surgeon at an HVC ($P<.05$) and more likely to receive care at LVCs by low-volume surgeons, increasing the disparity gap in outcomes and survival. Wasif and colleagues[71] also found that Black patients were less likely to receive care at HVCs (OR 0.83, CI 0.74–0.92); similarly, uninsured patients and those residing in zip codes with lower population-level educational attainment were also unlikely to receive care at HVCs.

Geography also plays a significant role in access to cancer care,[19,66,67,72] and in this regard, regionalization of care has negatively impacted outcomes by creating a geographic barrier to health care access. Several studies have reported worse survival, worse quality of life, more complications, and higher readmission rates in patients with longer travel distances to sites of treatment.[73–75] O'Connor and colleagues[76] highlighted the association of longer travel distances and decreased overall survival in patients with extrahepatic biliary tumors. Patients who traveled longer distances to receive care have also been shown to have lower median household incomes, further amplifying the barriers to care surrounding patients' ability to afford travel, to request time off from work, and to coordinate multiple trips for therapy.[15] In addition, zip code of residence is associated with receipt of surgery at HVCs,[77] and rural residence has been associated with lower medical and radiation oncology consultation rates.[77–80]

Access to care at HVCs is associated with improved surgical outcomes and increased access to multimodality therapy, both of which are associated with improved survival in the treatment of PC. However, access to these HVCs is inequitable, thus further perpetuating disparate survival for PC between White and BIPOC patients. Ensuring equitable access to HVCs will require addressing nonmedical social determinants of health, such as inequities in education, labor, housing markets, and exposure to the criminal justice system.

UNDERREPRESENTATION IN CLINICAL TRIALS

Despite the National Comprehensive Cancer Network recommendation for patients with cancer to enroll in clinical trials, only 2% to 4% of patients participate.[81] Underrepresented minorities only comprise 15% of patients enrolled in clinical trials, with significant underrepresentation from Black, Hispanic, and elderly patients, raising concerns over access to participation in trials.[82,83] Zaorsky and colleagues[81] found patients who enrolled in clinical trials were more likely to be White, have metastatic disease, be privately insured, have fewer comorbidities, and, somewhat surprisingly, live farther away from the treatment center than those who did not participate. The preceding findings suggest that access to health insurance and hospitals that participate in clinical trials are barriers to enrollment of minorities, but that physical distance to treating hospitals, in and of itself, is not. Several studies exploring racial barriers to clinical trial enrollment highlight historical discrimination toward minority groups, with concomitantly decreased trust in the health care system, entrenched concerns regarding exploitation, and perceived nontransparency regarding treatment and researcher motivation on the part of minorities.[82,84,85] Large clinical trials provide the best level of evidence to guide treatment decisions; however, when trials do not include and represent a diverse patient population, physicians must question if the data have real-world applicability. To decrease the disparity in outcomes of patients with cancer, efforts to increase minority participation in clinical trials and to address the multiple aforementioned factors contributing to this disparity must be addressed.

SUMMARY

In summary, incidence, presentation, biology, treatment opportunities, and outcomes in PC vary tremendously across the spectrum of patients. Race, gender, ethnicity, geography, and socioeconomic factors can affect each of these, and inequities related to any of these factors can lead to late presentation, undertreatment, and poor outcomes (**Fig. 1**). In a deadly disease such as PC, these inequities are amplified and lead to significantly worse outcomes in our most vulnerable populations. Awareness of these trends and factors provides the first step toward correcting these disparities and ultimately providing just, culturally competent, and equitable care for all patients with PC.

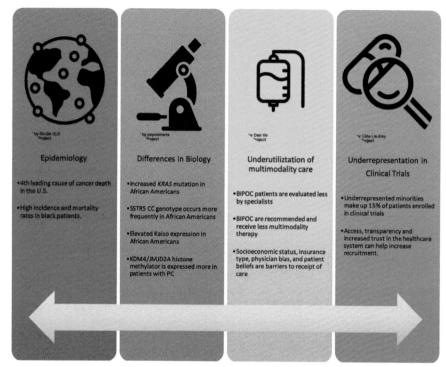

Fig. 1. Factors that contribute to the undertreatment of PC.

DISCLOSURE

The authors have nothing to disclose.

REFERENCES

1. Siegel RL, Miller KD, Fuchs HE, et al. Cancer statistics, 2021. CA Cancer J Clin 2021;71(1):7–33.

2. Rahib L, Smith BD, Aizenberg R, et al. Projecting cancer incidence and deaths to 2030: the unexpected burden of thyroid, liver, and pancreas cancers in the United States. Cancer Res 2014;74(11):2913–21.

3. Grossberg AJ, Chu LC, Deig CR, et al. Multidisciplinary standards of care and recent progress in pancreatic ductal adenocarcinoma. CA Cancer J Clin 2020; 70(5):375–403.

4. Prakash O, Hossain F, Danos D, et al. Racial disparities in triple negative breast cancer: a review of the role of biologic and non-biologic factors. Front Public Health 2020;8:576964.

5. Yao S, Cheng TD, Elkhanany A, et al. Breast tumor microenvironment in black women: a distinct signature of CD8+ T cell exhaustion. J Natl Cancer Inst 2021. https://doi.org/10.1093/jnci/djaa215.

6. Mitchell KA, Zingone A, Toulabi L, et al. Differences in NSCLC from African Americans and European Americans. Clin Cancer Res 2017;23(23):7412–25.

7. Buscail L, Bournet B, Cordelier P. Role of oncogenic KRAS in the diagnosis, prognosis and treatment of pancreatic cancer. Nat Rev Gastroenterol Hepatol 2020; 17(3):153–68.

8. Pernick NL, Sarkar FH, Philip PA, et al. Clinicopathologic analysis of pancreatic adenocarcinoma in African Americans and Caucasians. Pancreas 2003;26(1): 28–32.

9. Ward E, Jemal A, Cokkinides V, et al. Cancer disparities by race/ethnicity and socioeconomic status. CA Cancer J Clin 2004;54(2):78–93.

10. Bailey ZD, Krieger N, Agénor M, et al. Structural racism and health inequities in the USA: evidence and interventions. Lancet 2017;389(10077):1453–63.

11. Collin LJ, Gaglioti AH, Beyer KM, et al. Neighborhood-level redlining and lending bias are associated with breast cancer mortality in a large and diverse metropolitan area. Cancer Epidemiol Biomarkers Prev 2021;30(1):53–60.

12. based on November 2019 SEER data submission, posted to the SEER. In: Howlader NNA, Krapcho M, Miller D, et al, editors. SEER cancer statistics review, 1975-2017. Bethesda, MD: National Cancer Institute; 2020. Available at: https://seer.cancer.gov/csr/1975_2017/ https://seer.cancer.gov/statistics/. Accessed February 15, 2021.

13. Lim JE, Chien MW, Earle CC. Prognostic factors following curative resection for pancreatic adenocarcinoma: a population-based, linked database analysis of 396 patients. Ann Surg 2003;237(1):74–85.

14. Fesinmeyer MD, Austin MA, Li CI, et al. Differences in survival by histologic type of pancreatic cancer. Cancer Epidemiol Biomarkers Prev 2005;14(7):1766–73.

15. Bach PB, Schrag D, Brawley OW, et al. Survival of blacks and whites after a cancer diagnosis. JAMA 2002;287(16):2106–13.

16. Silverman DT, Hoover RN, Brown LM, et al. Why do Black Americans have a higher risk of pancreatic cancer than White Americans? Epidemiology 2003; 14(1):45–54.

17. Brotherton L, Welton M, Robb SW. Racial disparities of pancreatic cancer in Georgia: a county-wide comparison of incidence and mortality across the state, 2000-2011. Cancer Med 2016;5(1):100–10.

18. Arnold LD, Patel AV, Yan Y, et al. Are racial disparities in pancreatic cancer explained by smoking and overweight/obesity? Cancer Epidemiol Biomarkers Prev 2009;18(9):2397–405.

19. Network NCC. Pancreatic Adenocarcinoma (Version 2.2021). Available at: https://www.nccn.org/professionals/physician_gls/pdf/pancreatic.pdf. Accessed March 10, 2021.

20. Eheman C, Henley SJ, Ballard-Barbash R, et al. Annual report to the nation on the status of cancer, 1975-2008, featuring cancers associated with excess weight and lack of sufficient physical activity. Cancer 2012;118(9):2338–66.

21. Riner AN, Underwood PW, Yang K, et al. Disparities in pancreatic ductal adenocarcinoma-the significance of hispanic ethnicity, subgroup analysis, and treatment facility on clinical outcomes. Cancer Med 2020;9(12):4069–82.

22. Greenbaum A, Alkhalili E, Rodriguez R, et al. Pancreatic adenocarcinoma in New Mexico Native Americans: disparities in treatment and survival. J Health Care Poor Underserved 2019;30(2):609–17.

23. Siegel RL, Miller KD, Jemal A. Cancer statistics, 2015. CA Cancer J Clin 2015; 65(1):5–29.

24. Chang KJ, Parasher G, Christie C, et al. Risk of pancreatic adenocarcinoma: disparity between African Americans and other race/ethnic groups. Cancer 2005;103(2):349–57.

25. Nagata Y, Abe M, Motoshima K, et al. Frequent glycine-to-aspartic acid mutations at codon 12 of c-Ki-ras gene in human pancreatic cancer in Japanese. Jpn J Cancer Res 1990;81(2):135–40.

26. Song MM, Nio Y, Dong M, et al. Comparison of K-ras point mutations at codon 12 and p21 expression in pancreatic cancer between Japanese and Chinese patients. J Surg Oncol 2000;75(3):176–85.

27. Vick AD, Hery DN, Markowiak SF, et al. Closing the disparity in pancreatic cancer outcomes: a closer look at nonmodifiable factors and their potential use in treatment. Pancreas 2019;48(2):242–9.

28. Li D, Tanaka M, Brunicardi FC, et al. Association between somatostatin receptor 5 gene polymorphisms and pancreatic cancer risk and survival. Cancer 2011; 117(13):2863–72.

29. Zhou G, Gingras MC, Liu SH, et al. The hypofunctional effect of P335L single nucleotide polymorphism on SSTR5 function. World J Surg 2011;35(8):1715–24.

30. Adkins RM, Krushkal J, Tylavsky FA, et al. Racial differences in gene-specific DNA methylation levels are present at birth. Birth Defects Res A Clin Mol Teratol 2011;91(8):728–36.

31. Jones J, Mukherjee A, Karanam B, et al. African Americans with pancreatic ductal adenocarcinoma exhibit gender differences in Kaiso expression. Cancer Lett 2016;380(2):513–22.

32. Isohookana J, Haapasaari KM, Soini Y, et al. KDM4D predicts recurrence in exocrine pancreatic cells of resection margins from patients with pancreatic adenocarcinoma. Anticancer Res 2018;38(4):2295–302.

33. He J, Schulick RD, Del Chiaro M. Landmark series: neoadjuvant treatment in borderline resectable pancreatic cancer. Ann Surg Oncol 2021;28(3):1514–20.

34. Mizrahi JD, Surana R, Valle JW, et al. Pancreatic cancer. Lancet 2020; 395(10242):2008–20.

35. Abraham A, Al-Refaie WB, Parsons HM, et al. Disparities in pancreas cancer care. Ann Surg Oncol 2013;20(6):2078–87.

36. Heller DR, Nicolson NG, Ahuja N, et al. Association of treatment inequity and ancestry with pancreatic ductal adenocarcinoma survival. JAMA Surg 2020; 155(2):e195047.

37. Bilimoria KY, Bentrem DJ, Ko CY, et al. National failure to operate on early stage pancreatic cancer. Ann Surg 2007;246(2):173–80.

38. Moaven O, Richman JS, Reddy S, et al. Healthcare disparities in outcomes of patients with resectable pancreatic cancer. Am J Surg 2019;217(4):725–31.

39. Riall TS, Townsend CM, Kuo YF, et al. Dissecting racial disparities in the treatment of patients with locoregional pancreatic cancer: a 2-step process. Cancer 2010; 116(4):930–9.

40. Shah A, Chao KS, Ostbye T, et al. Trends in racial disparities in pancreatic cancer surgery. J Gastrointest Surg 2013;17(11):1897–906.

41. Murphy MM, Simons JP, Hill JS, et al. Pancreatic resection: a key component to reducing racial disparities in pancreatic adenocarcinoma. Cancer 2009;115(17): 3979–90.

42. Sandroussi C, Brace C, Kennedy ED, et al. Sociodemographics and comorbidities influence decisions to undergo pancreatic resection for neoplastic lesions. J Gastrointest Surg 2010;14(9):1401–8.

43. Shapiro M, Chen Q, Huang Q, et al. Associations of socioeconomic variables with resection, stage, and survival in patients with early-stage pancreatic cancer. JAMA Surg 2016;151(4):338–45.

44. Murphy MM, Simons JP, Ng SC, et al. Racial differences in cancer specialist consultation, treatment, and outcomes for locoregional pancreatic adenocarcinoma. Ann Surg Oncol 2009;16(11):2968–77.
45. Khanal N, Upadhyay S, Dahal S, et al. Systemic therapy in stage IV pancreatic cancer: a population-based analysis using the National Cancer Data Base. Ther Adv Med Oncol 2015;7(4):198–205.
46. Sridhar P, Misir P, Kwak H, et al. Impact of race, insurance status, and primary language on presentation, treatment, and outcomes of patients with pancreatic adenocarcinoma at a safety-net hospital. J Am Coll Surg 2019;229(4):389–96.
47. Pérez-Stable EJ, Sabogal F, Otero-Sabogal R, et al. Misconceptions about cancer among Latinos and Anglos. JAMA 1992;268(22):3219–23.
48. Cheung MC, Yang R, Byrne MM, et al. Are patients of low socioeconomic status receiving suboptimal management for pancreatic adenocarcinoma? Cancer 2010;116(3):723–33.
49. Loehrer AP, Chang DC, Hutter MM, et al. Health insurance expansion and treatment of pancreatic cancer: does increased access lead to improved care? J Am Coll Surg 2015;221(6):1015–22.
50. Moskowitz GB, Stone J, Childs A. Implicit stereotyping and medical decisions: unconscious stereotype activation in practitioners' thoughts about African Americans. Am J Public Health 2012;102(5):996–1001.
51. Manfredi C, Kaiser K, Matthews AK, et al. Are racial differences in patient-physician cancer communication and information explained by background, predisposing, and enabling factors? J Health Commun 2010;15(3):272–92.
52. Johnson RL, Roter D, Powe NR, et al. Patient race/ethnicity and quality of patient-physician communication during medical visits. Am J Public Health 2004;94(12):2084–90.
53. Esnaola NF, Ford ME. Racial differences and disparities in cancer care and outcomes: where's the rub? Surg Oncol Clin North Am 2012;21(3):417–37, viii.
54. van Ryn M, Burke J. The effect of patient race and socio-economic status on physicians' perceptions of patients. Soc Sci Med 2000;50(6):813–28.
55. Gansler T, Henley SJ, Stein K, et al. Sociodemographic determinants of cancer treatment health literacy. Cancer 2005;104(3):653–60.
56. Eloubeidi MA, Desmond RA, Wilcox CM, et al. Prognostic factors for survival in pancreatic cancer: a population-based study. Am J Surg 2006;192(3):322–9.
57. Tohme S, Kaltenmeier C, Bou-Samra P, et al. Race and health disparities in patient refusal of surgery for early-stage pancreatic cancer: an NCDB Cohort Study. Ann Surg Oncol 2018;25(12):3427–35.
58. Musa D, Schulz R, Harris R, et al. Trust in the health care system and the use of preventive health services by older black and white adults. Am J Public Health 2009;99(7):1293–9.
59. Kennedy BR, Mathis CC, Woods AK. African Americans and their distrust of the health care system: healthcare for diverse populations. J Cult Divers 2007;14(2):56–60.
60. Lieberman MD, Kilburn H, Lindsey M, et al. Relation of perioperative deaths to hospital volume among patients undergoing pancreatic resection for malignancy. Ann Surg 1995;222(5):638–45.
61. Gordon TA, Burleyson GP, Tielsch JM, et al. The effects of regionalization on cost and outcome for one general high-risk surgical procedure. Ann Surg 1995;221(1):43–9.
62. Ho V, Heslin MJ. Effect of hospital volume and experience on in-hospital mortality for pancreaticoduodenectomy. Ann Surg 2003;237(4):509–14.

63. Gouma DJ, van Geenen RC, van Gulik TM, et al. Rates of complications and death after pancreaticoduodenectomy: risk factors and the impact of hospital volume. Ann Surg 2000;232(6):786–95.
64. Birkmeyer JD, Finlayson SR, Tosteson AN, et al. Effect of hospital volume on in-hospital mortality with pancreaticoduodenectomy. Surgery 1999;125(3):250–6.
65. Birkmeyer JD, Siewers AE, Finlayson EV, et al. Hospital volume and surgical mortality in the United States. N Engl J Med 2002;346(15):1128–37.
66. Bilimoria KY, Bentrem DJ, Ko CY, et al. Multimodality therapy for pancreatic cancer in the U.S. : utilization, outcomes, and the effect of hospital volume. Cancer 2007;110(6):1227–34.
67. La Torre M, Nigri G, Ferrari L, et al. Hospital volume, margin status, and long-term survival after pancreaticoduodenectomy for pancreatic adenocarcinoma. Am Surg 2012;78(2):225–9.
68. Bliss LA, Yang CJ, Chau Z, et al. Patient selection and the volume effect in pancreatic surgery: unequal benefits? HPB (Oxford) 2014;16(10):899–906.
69. Al-Refaie WB, Muluneh B, Zhong W, et al. Who receives their complex cancer surgery at low-volume hospitals? J Am Coll Surg 2012;214(1):81–7.
70. Epstein AJ, Gray BH, Schlesinger M. Racial and ethnic differences in the use of high-volume hospitals and surgeons. Arch Surg 2010;145(2):179–86.
71. Wasif N, Etzioni D, Habermann EB, et al. Racial and socioeconomic differences in the use of high-volume commission on cancer-accredited hospitals for cancer surgery in the United States. Ann Surg Oncol 2018;25(5):1116–25.
72. Sinding C, Warren R, Fitzpatrick-Lewis D, et al. Research in cancer care disparities in countries with universal healthcare: mapping the field and its conceptual contours. Support Care Cancer 2014;22(11):3101–20.
73. Etzioni DA, Fowl RJ, Wasif N, et al. Distance bias and surgical outcomes. Med Care 2013;51(3):238–44.
74. Stitzenberg KB, Chang Y, Smith AB, et al. Exploring the burden of inpatient readmissions after major cancer surgery. J Clin Oncol 2015;33(5):455–64.
75. Scoggins JF, Fedorenko CR, Donahue SM, et al. Is distance to provider a barrier to care for Medicaid patients with breast, colorectal, or lung cancer? J Rural Health 2012;28(1):54–62.
76. O'Connor SC, Mogal H, Russell G, et al. The effects of travel burden on outcomes after resection of extrahepatic biliary malignancies: results from the US extrahepatic biliary consortium. J Gastrointest Surg 2017;21(12):2016–24.
77. Eppsteiner RW, Csikesz NG, McPhee JT, et al. Surgeon volume impacts hospital mortality for pancreatic resection. Ann Surg 2009;249(4):635–40.
78. Dumbrava MI, Burmeister EA, Wyld D, et al. Chemotherapy in patients with unresected pancreatic cancer in Australia: a population-based study of uptake and survival. Asia Pac J Clin Oncol 2018;14(4):326–36.
79. Johnston GM, Boyd CJ, Joseph P, et al. Variation in delivery of palliative radiotherapy to persons dying of cancer in Nova Scotia, 1994 to 1998. J Clin Oncol 2001;19(14):3323–32.
80. Yee EK, Coburn NG, Davis LE, et al. Impact of geography on care delivery and survival for noncurable pancreatic adenocarcinoma: a population-based analysis. J Natl Compr Canc Netw 2020;18(12):1642–50.
81. Zaorsky NG, Zhang Y, Walter V, et al. Clinical trial accrual at initial course of therapy for cancer and its impact on survival. J Natl Compr Canc Netw 2019;17(11):1309–16.
82. Murthy VH, Krumholz HM, Gross CP. Participation in cancer clinical trials: race-, sex-, and age-based disparities. JAMA 2004;291(22):2720–6.

83. Stewart JH, Bertoni AG, Staten JL, et al. Participation in surgical oncology clinical trials: gender-, race/ethnicity-, and age-based disparities. Ann Surg Oncol 2007; 14(12):3328–34.
84. Corbie-Smith G, Thomas SB, Williams MV, et al. Attitudes and beliefs of African Americans toward participation in medical research. J Gen Intern Med 1999; 14(9):537–46.
85. Shavers-Hornaday VL, Lynch CF, Burmeister LF, et al. Why are African Americans under-represented in medical research studies? Impediments to participation. Ethn Health 1997;2(1-2):31–45.

Disparities in Clinical Trial Participation

Multilevel Opportunities for Improvement

Brooke A. Stewart[a], John H. Stewart IV, MD, MBA[b,c,*]

KEYWORDS

- Surgical oncology • Clinical trials • Health equity • Implicit bias • Patient navigation
- Health policy

KEY POINTS

- Current data demonstrate ongoing inequities in surgical oncology clinical trials and understanding these disparities is vital to creating a more just and equitable health care system.
- The underlying causes of the inequities in participatory patterns in surgical oncology clinical trials are complex and require analysis at the levels of the patient, the provider, and the health care system.
- Holistic approaches to addressing disparities in clinical trial participation include creating a more robust pipeline of minority surgeon-scientists, engaging in partnerships with community advocates, and promoting public policy that addresses barriers to the recruitment and retention of minority patients in clinical trials.

INTRODUCTION

Cancer therapies have advanced substantially in recent years, but racial and ethnic minority groups in the United States have benefited less from those advances than their White counterparts. This disparity in outcomes results from the fact that race and ethnicity continue to shape access to important health care resources in the United States including clinical trials. Although the conduct of inclusive clinical trials is the only proven strategy for proving the safety of new cancer treatments and for improving the standard of care, less than 5% of all eligible adult patients enroll in oncology clinical trials.[1,2] The gains in trial participation in the period immediately after the passage of the National Institutes of Health (NIH) Revitalization Act of 1993 were seen primarily in the accrual of White males. The ongoing underrepresentation in trials represents a continuing inequity in health care in the United States as only about 14% of oncology clinical trial enrollees are members of minority populations.[2]

[a] Department of Psychology, Appalachian State University, Boone, NC, USA; [b] Louisiana State University, New Orleans School of Medicine; [c] Louisiana State University New Orleans- Louisiana Children's Medical Center Cancer Center, New Orleans, Louisiana, USA
* Corresponding author. Louisiana State University, New Orleans School of Medicine.
E-mail address: Jste17@lsuhsc.edu

Surg Oncol Clin N Am 31 (2022) 55–64
https://doi.org/10.1016/j.soc.2021.07.007
1055-3207/22/© 2021 Elsevier Inc. All rights reserved.

Understanding disparities in clinical trial participation is vital to creating a more just and equitable health care system. The exclusion of underrepresented groups from clinical trials jeopardizes the generalization of the results of these trials. Ensuring diverse participation in clinical trials will lead to more robust data that benefits all populations.[3] Moreover, the inclusion of minority patients in clinical trials may not only represent an important component of addressing disparities in outcome, but it might also improve the *delivery* of health care services to these populations.

Here, we review current participatory patterns in surgical oncology trials and describe the disparities that have been observed over time. We propose patient-, provider-, and policy-level interventions and community-centered solutions to stimulate trial participation among diverse patients.

THE CURRENT STATE OF PARTICIPATION IN SURGICAL ONCOLOGY CLINICAL TRIALS

A few trials have specifically evaluated the participation of minority groups in surgical oncology clinical trials, that is, trials for oncology patients in which a surgical intervention was being studied and/or surgery was required for inclusion. It is important to understand their findings to develop potential strategies to address clinical trial inequities.

Newman and colleagues undertook a retrospective study of patients registered on American College of Surgeons Oncology Group (ACOSOG) breast, thoracic, and colorectal clinical trials to evaluate accrual patterns for patients participating in the cancer protocols. The authors reported that the average accrual of African-American participants was 7.4%, including 5.7% for the thoracic studies, 8.6% for the breast studies, and 11.6% for the colorectal studies. On the contrary, the accrual of non-White Hispanic patients was 2.2%, including 0.6% for the thoracic studies, 3.7% for the breast studies, and 5.8% for the colorectal studies. The enrollment levels of African-American and Hispanic patients in ACOSOG trials were similar to the burden of cancer in these populations. Although the accrual of minority patients to the ACOSOG thoracic trials appeared notably lower, this difference disappeared after adjustments for trial eligibility criteria.[4]

Diehl and colleagues compared participation of African-American and Hispanic patients in 10 ACOSOG breast, sarcoma, and thoracic trials against accrual targets derived from both general population demographics and estimates of the distribution of racial/ethnic minorities within specific cancer types, stratified by stage. They reported that 8 of 10 trials were successful or modestly successful with regard to recruitment of African-American and/or Hispanic-American participants; only one trial (Breast Z1031) was successful in recruiting both African-American (15%) and Hispanic-American (13%) patients, whereas thoracic trials Z0030 and Z0060 were unsuccessful in recruiting both African-American and Hispanic-American participants. The authors also identified that clinical trials that were limited to regional or advanced-stage disease and those that involved some investigational systemic therapy approaches were the most successful in recruiting diverse study populations.[5]

Stewart and colleagues reviewed participatory patterns in National Cancer Institute (NCI)-sponsored surgical oncology trials for breast, prostate, lung, and colorectal cancer. This retrospective study evaluated the characteristics of 13,991 patients from the Cancer Therapeutic Evaluation Program (CTEP) Surgical Oncology Trial Database and found that 86.57% of trial participants were White, 7.92% were African-American, 3.4% were Hispanic, and 1.86% were Asian/Pacific islanders. The authors compared patient-level characteristics to estimated US cancer cases by race and histology. The primary outcome measure of enrollment was the enrollment fraction (EF), which was defined as the number of trial participants divided by incident cancer cases in the population.[1] The authors found that African-American and Hispanic patients were underrepresented in surgical trials relative to their proportion of incident cancers over the 3-year study period. Compared with White patients (EF, 0.72%), lower EFs were noted in African-American (0.48%; odds ratio [OR], 0.67; P < .001), Hispanic (0.54%, OR 0.76, P < .001), and Asian/Pacific Islander (0.59%; OR, 0.82; P = .001) patients. When stratified by tumor site, African-Americans, Hispanics, and Asian/Pacific Islanders were less likely to enroll in surgical trials for breast cancer than White patients. Interestingly, Hispanic patients were more likely to participate in surgical trials for colorectal cancer than their White counterparts (0.30%; OR, 1.54; P = .002), whereas African-Americans were significantly less likely to participate in colorectal cancer trials than their White counterparts (0.13%; OR, 0.64; P = .001). Based on these findings, the authors concluded that strategies to increase accrual to surgical trials and ameliorate disparities related to race/ethnicity, gender, and age were needed.[6]

Fayanju et al. recently evaluated zip code-level data from the National Cancer Database (NCDB) and patients included in the CTEP Surgical Oncology Trial Database to identify population-level determinants of participation in breast surgical oncology trials from 2000 to 2012. This study found that area-based patient income was strongly associated with clinical trial participation but in varying ways and to different extents across racial and ethnic groups. Overall, patients from the highest area-based income bracket (>$63,000) were less likely to participate than those from the lowest income bracket (<$38,000: OR, 0.63; 95% confidence interval [CI], 0.59–0.68), and the likelihood of enrollment declined with increasing income (P < .001). Although the likelihood of trial enrollment declined for all racial and ethnic groups over time because of overall decrease in trial size and concomitantly fewer opportunities for enrollment, there were statistically significant differences *within* racial/ethnic and income groups. In 2000 to 2003, when trial participation was the highest across all groups, Asian/Pacific Islander (7.17%), Hispanic (3.48%), and White (7.13%) patients from the highest income group (>$63,000) had greater trial participation than their counterparts in the lowest income group (<$38,000; Asian/Pacific Islander = 3.95%, Hispanic = 2.67%, White = 5.96%; P = .003). However, by 2008 to 2012, participation had fallen drastically for all races and ethnicities and only White high-income patients had a higher unadjusted participation rate than their lower-income counterparts (0.32% vs 0.25%; P < .001). Interestingly, trial participation was higher among low-income Black patients than high-income Black patients in 2000 to 2003 (5.56% vs 4.45%) and 2004 to 2007 (2.59% vs 1.89%), but these rates were equal by 2008 to 2012 (0.35% for both income groups).[7] The authors concluded that these intraracial differences in participation by income level highlighted the importance of appreciating the diversity *within* each racial/ethnic group and the need to use multifaceted strategies to mitigate observed disparities in trial participation across traditionally underrepresented groups.

BARRIERS TO PARTICIPATION IN CLINICAL TRIALS

Barriers to participation in clinical trials are multifactorial and include challenges at the level of patients (eg, mistrust of the medical system), providers (eg, implicit bias), and the US health care system (eg, lack of diversity among clinical trial investigators).

Mistrust of the medical system has been suggested as an underlying cause of unequal enrollment in clinical trials. The role of medical mistrust in the decision-making process of patients is complex. The medical establishment has a long history of mistreatment toward African-Americans, ranging from experiments on enslaved people to forced sterilizations of Black women to the denial of available, life-saving treatment to Black men in the Tuskegee Syphilis Study. There is, however, evidence that minority patients are willing to participate in clinical trials if the opportunity is presented to them. Wendler and colleagues reviewed 20 trials that reported the enrollment decisions of more than 70,000 patients to evaluate the claim that racial and ethnic minorities are less willing to participate in clinical trials. There was no difference between African-Americans and their White counterparts with regards to clinical trial enrollment in the 10 interventional studies included in this analysis (45.3% vs 41.8%; OR, 1.06; 95% CI, 0.78–1.45). Likewise, there was no statistically significant difference in the overall consent rate between Black and White patients in the 7 surgical trials included in this investigation (65.8% vs 47.8%; OR, 1.26; 95% CI, 0.89–1.77).[8] A more recent study of clinical trial participation demonstrated that African-American (OR, 1.40; 95% CI, 1.09–1.79; P = .0078) and Hispanic patients (OR, 1.84; 95% CI, 1.35–2.50; P = .0001) are more likely to participate in clinical trials than their White counterparts.[9] These findings contradict the widely held belief that patients of color are less willing to participate in surgical clinical trials.

The discussion of all treatment options is the foundation of the ethical shared decision-making in oncology. Likewise, a balanced presentation of clinical trials significantly influences a patient's decision to consider enrolling in them.[10,11] An understanding of how health care providers engage in clinical trial recruitment may provide insights into ways to improve the recruitment of diverse populations into surgical oncology clinical trials. As previously mentioned, recent studies have shown that most patients would participate in clinical trials if they were proposed to them.[4] However, physicians may be more reluctant to present clinical trials to minority patients due to implicit bias.[12,13] Implicit bias, which refers to stereotypes and attitudes that affect decision-making, understanding, and ultimately actions in an unconscious manner, has been shown to impact patient-provider interactions and subsequently lead to treatment decisions that exacerbate health care disparities.[14,15] Niranjan and colleagues evaluated health care providers' and clinical research professionals' perceptions of minority patients and found that many in these groups held negative stereotypes of minority patients including noncompliance and low health literacy.[12] Implicit bias also clouds providers' perceptions of comorbidity in potential trial participants. Comorbidities including cerebrovascular and cardiovascular diseases disproportionately affect minority patients. These conditions also, however, frequently disqualify patients from participation in clinical trials, thereby exacerbating disparities in clinical trial participation.[16] The impact of decisions on trial eligibility made at the intersection of implicit bias and comorbidity assessment is well-documented in an evaluation of patients with lung cancer by Lathan and colleagues Their study of 386 patients who met full eligibility for lung cancer surgery sought to explore factors that influence the receipt of lung cancer surgery. The authors reported that African-American patients with more than 2 comorbidities were found to be less likely to undergo lung cancer surgery than African-American patients with fewer than 2 comorbidities (OR, 0.04; 95% CI, 0.01–0.25). However, within the same cohort, White patients with extensive comorbidities were no less likely than their White counterparts with fewer comorbidities to undergo lung cancer surgery (OR, 0.45; 95% CI, 0.10–2.00). These findings suggest that implicit bias plays a significant role in the consideration of patients for inclusion in clinical trials.[15]

Broad ethnic representation among the leadership and general membership of a clinical trials cooperative group can improve the attention to ethnic and cultural inclusivity with which clinical trial protocols are designed, implemented, and ultimately applied to clinical practice. Greater diversity among physicians may also inspire more trust in ethnically diverse patient populations. Newman and colleagues considered this important topic in the context of ACOSOG clinical trials by reviewing the demographics of ACOSOG membership. They found a predominance of White American male surgeons (73%), a pattern that is seen in the overall physician workforce in the United States. Two percent of the ACOSOG surgeon-investigators identified as African-American, which was similar to the representation of Hispanic-American individuals.[4]

Given that academically oriented physicians are more likely to have the resources and motivation to enroll patients in clinical trials, arguably the most effective approach to demolishing provider- and practice-level barriers is addressing the professional pipeline of clinical trialists. Unfortunately, the pipeline for diverse surgeon-scientists is broken. Although African-Americans constitute 12.5% of the US population, they represented only 7.1% of the 2018 to 2019 medical school matriculants.[17] Concomitantly, having a small number of Black medical students impacts the applicant pool for residency training in surgical specialties. A recent review of data from the American Association of Medical Colleges (AAMC) showed that Blacks comprise only 4.5% of all surgical residents, and not surprisingly, Black faculty comprise only 4.2% of surgical faculty, a very small pool from which to cultivate surgeon-scientists who can lead surgical trials.[18]

Future work must use specific tactics that not only increase the number of minority health care professionals but also use targeted interventions that will increase the pool of minority surgical trialists. Diversity in the clinical research workforce catalyzes the scientific inquiry needed to tackle population-specific health issues experienced by vulnerable populations. We must find ways to strengthen the pipeline of surgical trainees from underrepresented groups into research careers that directly enhance equity in surgical oncology trials. Unfortunately, inadequate support in the clinical research career pipeline creates uphill barriers for trainees and contributes to disparities in the representation of investigators from underserved populations. Rather than waiting to support individuals from diverse backgrounds at later stages of the clinical research career path, when attrition has already reduced the talent pool, it is essential to provide early career development support and opportunities including research immersion for surgical trainees. Furthermore, these efforts must extend into and beyond undergraduate and graduate medical education. We call on the NCI to fund T32 training grants focused on underrepresented minority trainees in surgical oncology. This will allow for recruitment and cultivation of a cadre of surgeons who are appropriately trained to conduct clinical trials that are responsive to the needs of underserved communities.

HOLISTIC APPROACHES TO ELIMINATING INEQUITIES IN SURGICAL ONCOLOGY CLINICAL TRIALS

Community engagement, clinical trial navigation, and advocacy to promote public policy that eliminates the barriers to participation in surgical oncology trial will produce sustainable change in the access to and enrollment in these trials.

The "Community-To-Clinic" Model as an Approach to Sustainable Collaboration

Surgical trials must have an intentional focus on addressing the intersectionality of health at the individual, population, and environmental levels. Although the emphasis on a "bench-to-bedside" approach to clinical trials has arguably generated much success over the past 50 years, a gap clearly exists in bringing many of these investigations to underserved populations in an equitable manner. Indeed, a focus on this segment of the pathway to innovation has had the unintended effect of *widening* disparities in access to surgical trials. Dr Harold Freemen identified the "discovery-to-delivery" disconnect as a key contributor to cancer inequities and highlighted the necessity of extending scientific discovery to the community.[19] Furthermore, emerging community advocacy groups are demanding a seat at the table in the design and execution of clinical trials that will have a meaningful and definitively positive impact on their communities.[20] Therefore, it is time that clinical investigations in surgical oncology go beyond the familiar, linear ideology of the "bench-to-bedside" model, which is inherently unidirectional and limited to those patients who are fortunate enough to have their participation in clinical investigation both solicited and welcomed, to a cyclical "community-to-clinic" model that more effectively resolves the disconnect between development of therapeutic innovations and delivering them to the communities they should serve.

Central to the "community-to-clinic" approach are patient and community advocates who are involved in the design of surgical trials that are relevant to their communities. These advocates serve as ambassadors to support enrollment into these trials by members of their social networks, and they also serve as partners in the critical dissemination of clinical trial findings to their communities. The recently launched NIH "All of Us" program, which aims to enroll one million individuals to develop a database that would be widely available to academic research centers and the public at large, is an example of bridge-building between the "clinic" and the community.[21,22] It is a significant first step toward integrating community data into the conduct of scientific research and disseminating meaningful information back to the communities from which said data are sourced. This effort will require sustained intentionality to prioritize framing research with a focus on the individual and the communities in which they live, work, and play. Propelling the "community-to-clinic" model provides an opportunity to begin to mitigate the factors that contribute to disparities in clinical trial participation.

Clinical Trial Navigation to Address Barriers in Clinical Trial Enrollment

Given that the proportion of minority patients expressing a willingness to participate in a clinical trial is well above the proportion recruited into these trials, interventions that address social and logistical barriers such as transportation, life responsibilities, lack of insurance, and out-of-pocket expenses are warranted. Recent work by Meyers and colleagues has suggested that race alone is not a significant determinant of clinical trial participation, but rather that structural and financial barriers can and do preclude enrollment.[9] To that end, patient navigation programs have been adapted to address barriers to cancer trial participation among minority and medically underserved populations.[23] Patient navigation, a strategy for increasing patients' access to cancer care by helping them overcome barriers in their communities and within the health care system, was first described by Dr Harold Freeman to improve adherence to breast cancer care among African-American women.[24,25] Navigators serve as bridges between the patient and the health care system by providing education and facilitating the provision of services to the patient. As such, patient navigator training is fairly extensive and includes education and training on topics ranging from cancer care to cultural competency and ethics.[26–29]

Adapted from the patient navigator model, clinical trial navigators serve to increase participation through clinic-based education about clinical trials; thus, potential candidates would also require additional training in the principles of clinical trial design, human subjects research policies, and the counseling of potential participants on the risks and benefits of trial participation.[29] Clinical trial navigators can then provide support for patients based on an initial needs assessment. The support services provided by patient navigators already include assistance with visit logistics, appointment reminders, and referrals to social and community services and resources. In addition, clinical trial navigators can provide culturally appropriate peer support including accompanying patients to clinic visits when clinical trials will be discussed, offering social and emotional support, and serving as communication conduits for patients to report concerns to the research team. These strategies have been very successful in small studies that reported clinical trial enrollment between 61% and 86% among study-eligible minority patients.[30–32] With regard to participant retention, the investigators of the Increasing Minority Participation in Clinical Trials (IMPACT) reported a 74.5% trial retention and completion rate for patients who received clinical navigation compared with 37.5% for those who did not receive navigation support ($P < .001$).[33] We await the completion of a randomized trial to assess the effect of clinical trial navigators on enrollment into therapeutic cancer clinical trials.[34]

Advocacy as a Means to Increase Access to Clinical Trials

Advocacy in addressing health care policy issues will be an essential component of eliminating inequities in surgical clinical trials, and recent legislation has been proposed to address barriers to access to clinical trials. The Henrietta Lacks Enhancing Cancer Research Act of 2020 was signed into law on January 5, 2021, and the Clinical Treatment Act of 2020 is currently under consideration.

The Henrietta Lacks Enhancing Cancer Research Act of 2020 ensures that all patients, especially those from communities of color, are fairly represented in clinical trials and ultimately receive the treatments that they deserve. This law requires that the Government Accountability Office (GAO) completes a study reviewing what actions Federal agencies have taken to address barriers to participation in federally funded cancer clinical trials among populations that have been traditionally underrepresented in such trials and to identify challenges related to implementing such actions. The law also requires that the GAO submits a report to Congress on the results of this study, including recommendations on potential changes in practices and policies to improve participation in such trials among the populations of interest. Many suggest that this review will open up opportunities for further funded considerations around these important issues.

Currently, only 15 states and Washington, D.C., require their Medicaid programs to cover costs associated with routine care in clinical trials. Unfortunately, there are 41 million Medicaid recipients in the resulting coverage gap, undoubtedly limiting these individuals' access to clinical trials. This gap has a tremendous impact on minority patients, as 32.9% of African-American and 30.0% of Hispanic nonelderly patients are covered by Medicaid.[35] Senator Richard Burr and Representative Ben Ray Lujan recently introduced the Clinical Treatment Act of 2020 (bills S. 4742 and H.R. 913, respectively). Both bills are aimed at amending title XIX of the Social Security Act to promote access to life-saving therapies for Medicaid enrollees by ensuring coverage of routine patient costs for items and services furnished in connection with participation in qualifying clinical trials.

SUMMARY

The work contained herein lays a foundation for understanding disparities in surgical oncology clinical trial participation. Unequal enrollment persists, and the underlying causes for this inequity include implicit bias by providers and lack of diversity among clinical trial investigators. Sustainable change in clinical trial participation requires a holistic approach in which community members are engaged in the design of clinical trials and the dissemination of trial findings. Furthermore, all members of the research community must advocate for public policy that eliminates barriers to participation in the research process, thereby increasing access to trials for all patients. Finally, using clinical trial navigators to overcome local and systemic barriers to surgical oncology clinical trial participation will facilitate the recruitment and retention of diverse patients.

CLINICS CARE POINTS

- Current evidence demonstrates that distrust of the medical system is not a driver of lower rates of participation in surgical oncology trials among minority patients.

- Implicit bias has been shown to impact patient-provider interactions and subsequently lead to treatment decisions that exacerbate health care disparities. Implicit bias impacts all facets of the clinical investigation including trial design and the provider's willingness to discuss clinical trials with minority patients.

- Broad racial and ethnic representation among the leadership and general membership of a clinical trials group can improve the ethnic and cultural sensitivity of the protocols from the time of study design through the implementation and interpretation phases.

- Resolving differences in surgical oncology clinical trials will require a holistic approach that is founded on cooperation between relevant stakeholders. The "community-to-clinic model" in which patient and community advocates are involved in the design of surgical trials relevant to their communities is an excellent example of inclusive clinical trial partnership.

- Patient navigation programs have addressed barriers to cancer trial participation among minority and medically underserved populations. Patient navigation addresses barriers to clinical trial participation including transportation, lack of insurance, and out-of-pocket expenses.

DISCLOSURE

The authors have nothing to disclose.

REFERENCES

1. Murthy VH, Krumholz HM, Gross CP. Participation in cancer clinical trials: race-, sex-, and age-based disparities. JAMA 2004;291(22):2720–6.
2. Duma N, Vera Aguilera J, Paludo J, et al. Representation of minorities and women in oncology clinical trials: review of the past 14 years. J Oncol Pract 2018;14(1):e1–10.
3. Clark LT, Watkins L, Piña IL, et al. Increasing diversity in clinical trials: overcoming critical barriers. Curr Probl Cardiol 2019;44(5):148–72.
4. Newman LA, Hurd T, Leitch M, et al. A report on accrual rates for elderly and minority-ethnicity cancer patients to clinical trials of the American College of Surgeons Oncology Group. J Am Coll Surg 2004;199(4):644–51.
5. Diehl KM, Green EM, Weinberg A, et al. Features associated with successful recruitment of diverse patients onto cancer clinical trials: report from the American College of Surgeons Oncology Group. Ann Surg Oncol 2011;18(13):3544–50.
6. Stewart JH, Bertoni AG, Staten JL, et al. Participation in surgical oncology clinical trials: gender-, race/ethnicity-, and age-based disparities. Ann Surg Oncol 2007; 14(12):3328–34.
7. Fayanju OM, Ren Y, Thomas SM, et al. A case-control study examining disparities in clinical trial participation among breast surgical oncology patients. JNCI Cancer Spectr 2020;4(2):pkz103.

8. Wendler D, Kington R, Madans J, et al. Are racial and ethnic minorities less willing to participate in health research? PLoS Med 2006;3(2):e19.

9. Meyer S, Woldu HG, Sheets LR. Sociodemographic diversity in cancer clinical trials: New findings on the effect of race and ethnicity. Contemp Clin Trials Commun 2021;21:100718.

10. Leffall LD Jr. Claude H. Organ, Jr. Honorary/Sandoz Nutrition Lectureship. Ethics in research and surgical practice. Am J Surg 1997;174(6):589–91.

11. Leffall LD Jr. Ethics in surgical research. Surgery 1998;123(6):603–5.

12. Niranjan SJ, Martin MY, Fouad MN, et al. Bias and stereotyping among research and clinical professionals: perspectives on minority recruitment for oncology clinical trials. Cancer 2020;126(9):1958–68.

13. Chapman EN, Kaatz A, Carnes M. Physicians and implicit bias: how doctors may unwittingly perpetuate health care disparities. J Gen Intern Med 2013;28(11): 1504–10.

14. Sabin JA, Greenwald AG. The influence of implicit bias on treatment recommendations for 4 common pediatric conditions: pain, urinary tract infection, attention deficit hyperactivity disorder, and asthma. Am J Public Health 2012;102(5): 988–95.

15. Lathan CS, Neville BA, Earle CC. The effect of race on invasive staging and surgery in non-small-cell lung cancer. J Clin Oncol 2006;24(3):413–8.

16. Adams-Campbell LL, Ahaghotu C, Gaskins M, et al. Enrollment of African Americans onto clinical treatment trials: study design barriers. J Clin Oncol 2004;22(4): 730–4.

17. Colleges AAoM. 2019 fall applicant, matriculant, and enrollment data tables. 2019. Available at: https://www.aamc.org/system/files/2019-12/2019%20AAMC %20Fall%20Applicant. Accessed October 20, 2020.

18. Aggarwal A, Rosen CB, Nehemiah A, et al. Is there color or sex behind the mask and sterile blue? examining sex and racial demographics within academic surgery. Ann Surg 2021;273(1):21–7.

19. Freeman HP. Poverty, culture, and social injustice: determinants of cancer disparities. CA Cancer J Clin 2004;54(2):72–7.

20. Wallington SF, Dash C, Sheppard VB, et al. Enrolling minority and underserved populations in cancer clinical research. Am J Prev Med 2016;50(1):111–7.

21. Collins FS, Varmus H. A new initiative on precision medicine. N Engl J Med 2015; 372(9):793–5.

22. Sankar PL, Parker LS. The Precision Medicine Initiative's All of Us Research Program: an agenda for research on its ethical, legal, and social issues. Genet Med 2017;19(7):743–50.

23. Ghebre RG, Jones LA, Wenzel JA, et al. State-of-the-science of patient navigation as a strategy for enhancing minority clinical trial accrual. Cancer 2014;120 Suppl 7(0 7):1122–30.

24. Freeman HP, Muth BJ, Kerner JF. Expanding access to cancer screening and clinical follow-up among the medically underserved. Cancer Pract 1995;3(1): 19–30.

25. Paskett ED, Harrop JP, Wells KJ. Patient navigation: an update on the state of the science. CA Cancer J Clin 2011;61(4):237–49.

26. Petereit DG, Molloy K, Reiner ML, et al. Establishing a patient navigator program to reduce cancer disparities in the American Indian communities of Western South Dakota: initial observations and results. Cancer Control 2008;15(3):254–9.

27. Schapira L, Schutt R. Training community health workers about cancer clinical trials. J Immigr Minor Health 2011;13(5):891–8.

28. Bryant DC, Williamson D, Cartmell K, et al. A lay patient navigation training curriculum targeting disparities in cancer clinical trials. J Natl Black Nurses Assoc 2011;22(2):68–75.

29. Steinberg ML, Fremont A, Khan DC, et al. Lay patient navigator program implementation for equal access to cancer care and clinical trials: essential steps and initial challenges. Cancer 2006;107(11):2669–77.

30. Holmes DR, Major J, Lyonga DE, et al. Increasing minority patient participation in cancer clinical trials using oncology nurse navigation. Am J Surg 2012;203(4): 415–22.

31. Proctor JW, Martz E, Schenken LL, et al. A screening tool to enhance clinical trial participation at a community center involved in a radiation oncology disparities program. J Oncol Pract 2011;7(3):161–4.

32. Wujcik D, Wolff SN. Recruitment of African Americans to National Oncology Clinical Trials through a clinical trial shared resource. J Health Care Poor Underserved 2010;21(1 Suppl):38–50.

33. Fouad MN, Acemgil A, Bae S, et al. Patient navigation as a model to increase participation of African Americans in Cancer Clinical Trials. J Oncol Pract 2016; 12(6):556–63.

34. Uveges MK, Lansey DG, Mbah O, et al. Patient navigation and clinical trial participation: a randomized controlled trial design. Contemp Clin Trials Commun 2018; 12:98–102.

35. Foundation KF. Medicaid coverage for the nonelderly by race/ethnicity. 2021. Available at: https://www.kff.org/medicaid/state-indicator/nonelderly-medicaid-rate-by-raceethnicity/?currentTimeframe=0&sortModel=%7B%22colId%22:%22Location%22,%22sort%22:%22asc%22%7D. Accessed April 20, 2021.

Racial Disparities in the Management of Locoregional Colorectal Cancer

Scarlett Hao, MD, Alexander A. Parikh, MD, MPH,
Rebecca A. Snyder, MD, MPH*

KEYWORDS

- Disparities • Colorectal cancer • Surgery • Chemotherapy • Neoadjuvant
- Health policy

KEY POINTS

- Racial disparities exist in receipt of surgical resection, need for emergent resection, use of minimally invasive approaches, and adequacy of oncologic resection.
- Postoperative complications disproportionately affect Black patients.
- Receipt of multimodality therapy, including neoadjuvant radiation for rectal cancer and adjuvant chemotherapy for colon cancer, occurs at lower rates for patients from minority backgrounds.
- Survival and mortality outcomes are worse for Black patients.
- Successful disparity-targeted interventions approach modifiable factors on several levels.

INTRODUCTION

Despite decades of advances in preventative care and early detection, colorectal cancer (CRC) still ranks as one of the top four most common primary sites of cancer in the United States, with an estimated 149,500 new cases in 2021.[1] Incidence varies substantially by race, with the highest rates in patients of non-Hispanic Black race, followed by the American Indian/Alaskan Native (AI/AN) population.[2] The disparity gap in mortality is even wider, with death rates for Black patients almost 1.5 times that of non-Hispanic White patients (**Fig. 1**).[2] Evidence suggests that underlying etiologies for these disparities are broad and include socioeconomic disadvantage and lifestyle risk factors, disparities in screening, advanced stage at diagnosis, and differential receipt of treatment. This chapter specifically reviews current evidence on disparities in the treatment of locoregional CRC.

Division of Surgical Oncology, Department of Surgery, Brody School of Medicine at East Carolina University, 600 Moye Boulevard, Surgical Oncology Suite, 4S-24, Greenville, NC 27834, USA
* Corresponding author.
E-mail address: snyderre19@ecu.edu

Surg Oncol Clin N Am 31 (2022) 65–79
https://doi.org/10.1016/j.soc.2021.07.008
1055-3207/22/© 2021 Elsevier Inc. All rights reserved.

surgonc.theclinics.com

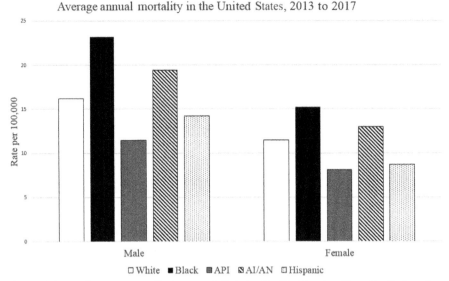

Average annual mortality in the United States, 2013 to 2017

Fig. 1. Colorectal cancer mortality by race. API, Asian/Pacific Islander. (*From* North American Association of Central Cancer Registries, 2020.)

TREATMENT

Unfortunately, despite recent advances in CRC treatment, not all patients have benefited equally.[3] Across all treatment modalities, patients of non-White race have a lower likelihood of receiving recommended treatment when compared with White patients.[4] In addition, the contribution of treatment disparities to the survival gap is significant.[5,6]

Time to Treatment Initiation

It has been clearly established that delay in initiation of CRC treatment correlates with worse survival outcomes.[7–9] In a multi-institutional study of 386 patients with colon cancer, low socioeconomic status (SES) and increased travel burden were associated with a prolonged delay to treatment initiation, and these factors disproportionately affected Black patients.[10] A study using the state of Georgia's registry data from 2010 to 2015 found an increased time to treatment, specifically increased time from diagnosis to surgery and from surgery to initiation of chemotherapy, among Black when compared with White patients with CRC.[11] On a national level, analyses of data from the Surveillance, Epidemiology, and End Results (SEER) program and the National Cancer Database (NCDB) have demonstrated that rates of delayed versus timely definitive surgical resection are highest among Black patients.[8] Interestingly, a study of patients treated for colon cancer within an equal access military health system found no differences in time to treatment between racial cohorts.[12]

Delays can also occur in the interval between surgical resection and initiation of adjuvant chemotherapy as a result of postoperative complications as well as patient age, comorbidity, and SES, although comprehensive studies on racial disparities of this metric are lacking.[13,14] Black patients with rectal cancer experience increased time from diagnosis to initiation of adjuvant chemoradiation (CRT), as well as longer time from completion of neoadjuvant CRT to surgical resection.[15] Although factors impacting time to treatment initiation vary, delays in cancer care, including colorectal surgery, have been exacerbated in the era of the COVID-19 pandemic.[16,17]

Surgery

Receipt of resection

Across multiple database studies, rates of surgical resection are consistently lower among Black compared with White patients with CRC, even among patients with early-stage disease.[11,18–20] Hispanic patients with CRC also have lower rates of resection compared with White patients.[18,21] In addition, for patients with rectal cancer, Black patients are more likely to receive nonoperative management.[22,23]

There are several reasons for the observed disparity in resection rates. Patients of minority race are often less likely to undergo surgery because of higher rates of significant comorbidity and later stage of disease at diagnosis. They may also be burdened by concurrent access-to-care barriers including forms of socioeconomic disadvantage such as inadequate insurance.[24] Available capabilities and technologies at smaller regional and critical-access hospitals are also a limiting factor for patients of minority race unable to seek care at large, resource-rich academic or comprehensive cancer centers.[11] Minority patients may also refuse surgery at higher rates compared with White patients.[25,26] And while not specifically studied in CRC care, both implicit bias and negative race-related beliefs held by providers likely play a role.[27,28]

Emergency surgery

Patients with CRC who require urgent or emergent resection have worse long-term outcomes, even when node-negative.[29,30] These include higher likelihood of recurrence, decreased disease-free survival, and worse overall survival.[31,32] Emergent resection is more often necessary in patients presenting with advanced disease,[29,33] which is more common in patients of minority race, although studies directly investigating the association of race with emergent resection are few. A SEER study found that Black patients had higher odds of undergoing emergency operations for CRC, which appeared to be compounded by an interaction effect of residence in high-poverty neighborhoods.[34] Efforts to reduce emergency presentation primarily center on increasing CRC screening.[33]

Oncologic adequacy of resection

Adequate oncologic resection for colon cancer requires a lymph node harvest of at least 12 nodes and negative resection margins.[35] Both metrics are associated with prognosis and survival outcomes and also inform decisions regarding adjuvant therapy. Literature on racial disparities in these metrics is limited. Data from Louisiana and California state registries, as well as the Department of Defense registry, suggest that Hispanic and Black patients are less likely to undergo an adequate lymphadenectomy, although this disparity did not fully correlate with or explain mortality outcomes.[36–38] In a study of 39,210 patients identified from the 1973 to 2006 SEER database, nodal counts did not differ between racial cohorts after multivariable adjustment, whereas survival did.[39] In contrast, a study of 2000 to 2003 SEER data suggested that Hispanic patients were less likely to undergo adequate lymph node resection but had equivalent survival to White patients.[40] Subtle differences in cohort selection and statistical analysis likely influenced the difference in findings between these 2 studies. A more recent NCDB study found equivalent rates of lymphadenectomy (defined as > 8 nodes) after neoadjuvant CRT for rectal cancer among White and Black patients, but again found a discrepancy in overall survival by race.[41] Thus, the data seem to suggest that racial disparities in nodal harvest exist but do not fully explain survival disparities. In addition, although positive resection margins strongly predict local recurrence, the interaction of margin status and race has not been investigated specifically in CRC.

Minimally invasive surgery

Minimally invasive surgery (MIS) including laparoscopic or robotic-assisted approaches offer potential benefits of reduced postoperative pain, decreased length of stay, and earlier advancement of diet/return of bowel function with noninferior oncologic outcomes.[42–44] However, not all patients are candidates for an MIS approach, particularly patients suffering from multiple comorbidities or with a history of prior abdominal operations.[43] In addition, access to MIS may also be limited by prohibitive cost.[45,46] Both clinical factors and financial limitations affect patients of minority race to a greater degree in general, but the literature on racial disparities in receipt of resection via MIS approach is conflicting.

Across 3 studies based on national data, race has generally not been found to be a significant factor influencing MIS approach for CRC.[45–47] However, 2 NCDB studies (2000–2012) found a lower likelihood of undergoing minimally invasive resection among Black patients with CRC, although in patients with rectal cancer, this racial disparity was only observed if patients were also uninsured.[47,48] More contemporary national trends—including rates of robotic resection—have not yet been reported.

Studies based on state or regional data sets suggest there are racial disparities in receipt of MIS. Within a single health system, Black and Asian patients were found to have a lower likelihood of undergoing colon resection via an MIS approach, although the study included benign and diverticular disease in addition to malignant indications.[49] An analysis of patients with CRC in the state of Florida found regional disparities for Hispanic patients receiving MIS, but this finding was not consistent across the entire state.[50] In addition, several of these studies document both socioeconomic factors and race as limiting the receipt of MIS, highlighting the intersection of race and socioeconomic disadvantage.[24]

Sphincter-sparing surgery

When oncologically feasible, sphincter-sparing surgery for the treatment of rectal cancer has less morbidity and noninferior oncologic outcomes compared with traditional abdominoperineal resection.[51] Retrospective data from the 1998 to 2006 Nationwide Inpatient Sample found that White patients are more likely to undergo sphincter-preserving surgery compared with Black and Hispanic patients.[52] This was redemonstrated on a more recent study using the same database.[53] The causes of this disparity remain unclear, however, and may be secondary to referral patterns, surgeon ability, physician biases, or tumor characteristics unfavorable to proceeding with sphincter-preserving surgery.

Postoperative complications

In patients who undergo surgical resection for CRC, postoperative complication rates may be higher among patients of minority race. Analysis of national data has demonstrated that Black patients undergoing resection for CRC experience higher rates of postoperative complications including in-hospital mortality, need for intensive care, increased length of stay, and increased readmission rates.[18,54,55] A study of benign and malignant colorectal surgery cases that specifically required small or large intestinal stoma creation using the 2013 to 2016 ACS NSQIP identified higher postoperative complication rates and prolonged hospital length of stay in patients of minority race.[56] More recent data in the era of enhanced recovery after surgery (ERAS) protocols are available but not specific to patients with cancer. Two studies found improved postsurgical outcomes after ERAS implementation for all patients without significant differences by race, an optimistic outcome that warrants investigation specifically in CRC patients.[57,58]

Radiation

Although surgery remains the mainstay of treatment in patients with resectable rectal cancer, there are proven benefits of neoadjuvant radiation in the locally advanced setting. Neoadjuvant radiation may allow for sphincter-sparing surgery in low rectal cancers and also decreases local recurrence.[59–61] National and single-institution data analyses have demonstrated greater likelihood of inadequate radiation dosing, as well as lower rates of neoadjuvant radiation, among Black patients with AJCC stage II and III rectal cancer.[62–64] Although an analysis of Florida state registry data found no association between race and receipt of radiation for rectal cancer, the use of neoadjuvant versus adjuvant radiation was not examined separately.[65] These disparities in guideline-concordant care warrant intervention.

Systemic Therapy

Colon

Randomized clinical trials have demonstrated a significant survival benefit of adjuvant systemic chemotherapy among patients with locoregional colon cancer.[66–69] Unfortunately, national data analyses have shown that Black patients with colon cancer are less likely to receive adjuvant systemic therapy.[20,70] Access to care for receipt of systemic therapy is likely impacted by the same barriers limiting receipt of surgical resection. A California registry study found that Black patients with colon cancer who are disadvantaged by both poverty and inadequate insurance experienced a disproportionately low rate of chemotherapy use compared with equally disadvantaged White patients.[71]

Despite indications that adjuvant chemotherapy in patients with stage III colon cancer improves survival, it remains underutilized.[72] In addition, analyses of SEER and NCDB data have found that Black patients with stage III disease are less likely to receive adjuvant chemotherapy compared with White patients.[73–75] Interestingly, a SEER Medicare study found that although Black patients with stage III colon cancer were less likely to initiate adjuvant chemotherapy, they were more likely to complete therapy compared to White patients treated with adjuvant chemotherapy.[74,76]

Emerging therapies including neoadjuvant systemic therapy (FOXTROT Collaborative) and immunotherapy in patients with microsatellite instability (A021502-ATOMIC) may have additional benefits to patients with locoregional CRC.[77,78] It will be essential to ensure that the implementation of new therapies or alternative treatment sequencing approaches does not lead to additional racial disparities.

Rectal

Guidelines support the use of systemic therapy in the management of locoregional rectal cancer.[79] However, as in colon cancer, Black patients with rectal cancer are less likely to receive systemic therapy.[80] An NCDB study on patients with stage II/III rectal cancer found low rates of receipt of adjuvant chemotherapy despite increased 5-year overall survival if given; this lack of adjuvant chemotherapy persisted on adjusted multivariable analyses for both Black and uninsured/underinsured patients.[81]

SURVIVAL OUTCOMES

Across multiple studies, Black patients with CRC experience higher rates of mortality and worse 5-year survival compared with White patients.[80,82–86] Evidence suggests this disparity is not mitigated by facility type.[87] Even with guideline-concordant care, Black patients have increased mortality compared with White patients, although the disparity is less pronounced when matched for treatment and stage.[6,88] Not surprisingly, survival disparities appear to be closely linked to treatment disparities as well as socioeconomic risk factors.[19]

Disease-Free Survival and Recurrence

Analyses of trial-enrolled patients with CRC—who one would presume all received the same treatment—have found increased risk of recurrence and decreased disease-free survival among Black patients.[89–91] Similar findings were noted in an NCDB study of patients who received guideline-concordant care for colon cancer.[88] In these studies, assumption of adequate treatment suggests alternative factors leading to the disparate rates of recurrence. A recent study found that Black patients were more likely to receive no post-treatment surveillance testing after resection of stage II/III colon cancer, suggesting an additional disparity of survivorship care for patients of minority race.[92]

Quality of Life and Patient-Reported Outcomes

Owing to advances in screening, diagnosis, and treatment for CRC, life expectancy of patients with CRC is improved; therefore, addressing the long-term effects of the disease as well as its treatment is critical. Most recent 5-year survival rates of all cases of CRC are over 65%.[93] In the survivorship phase of care, evaluation of health-related quality of life (HRQoL) is essential to guide counseling and management.[94] According to several studies, Black patients report worse physical and mental well-being on HRQoL assessments compared with White patients.[95,96] These differences are associated with worse overall survival.[95] Studies of Black patients with several cancer types including breast, lung, prostate, and colorectal have shown that social needs and financial hardship disproportionately affect Black cancer survivors and that these factors are associated with worse HRQoL.[97,98] Improvements in HRQoL disparities will depend on not only appropriate clinical support but also a concurrent focus on socioeconomic factors.

FUTURE DIRECTIONS
Other Racial Cohorts

To date, the literature on racial disparities in CRC care focuses predominantly on the experience of Black patients. Not only is it important to compare outcomes in racially diverse cohorts, but it is also essential that these cohorts receive individual attention.[99] Whereas some groups may share negative disparities with Black patients, such as AI/AN patients who undergo resection at lower rates,[100,101] others have countertrends, such as Asian American patients who appear to have improved postoperative outcomes and survival after resection of CRC.[39,99,102]

Early-Onset Colorectal Cancer

Incidence rates of CRC in patients under the age of 50 years have been increasing since the 1990s.[103] This has also been found to disproportionately affect patients of minority race. Black and Hispanic patients have a higher incidence of early-onset CRC in addition to presenting with later stages of disease.[104–108] Young-adult patients of minority race also experience lower rates of receipt of treatment with concomitantly worse survival outcomes.[104,107,109–111] Finally, despite increased genetic mutations in early-onset CRC, fewer Black patients with early-onset CRC are referred for genetic testing or counseling.[112] Although some guidelines on screening colonoscopy now recommend earlier screening for Black patients in response to the increasing incidence of early-onset CRC,[113] racial disparities will persist without intervention on health care access and other barriers impeding appropriate treatment for patients of minority race.

Health Policy Changes and Disparity-Targeted Interventions

There is no single solution to the challenge of eliminating racial disparities in cancer care. Racial disparity itself has many confounders. Although race is a fixed construct, patients of minority race are also affected by a multitude of modifiable factors including health insurance, financial insecurity, neighborhood poverty, and health literacy, among many others.[24,71,114] Clinical risk factors including obesity and tobacco use affect patients of non-White race to a higher degree,[24] and the subpopulation of cancer patients with low health literacy, low educational attainment, and low income consists disproportionately of Black patients.[115] Unfortunately, existing cancer registries, databases, and clinical trial data fail to collect meaningful data on these key confounders, instead relying on more general, surrogate markers of disparity.[116] Studies designed to identify the most critical modifiable factors of racial disparity will be needed to inform future interventions.

Health insurance coverage has been a prime target for interventions designed to reduce barriers to care. State health care reform measures influenced the development of the Affordable Care Act in 2010, with measurable impact on various aspects of patient care including care for patients with cancer.[117] After coverage expansion measures passed in 2006 in the state of Massachusetts, a marked increase in rates of resection for CRC was noted.[118] However, although minority patients are more likely to be uninsured or underinsured, evidence suggests that even matching for optimal insurance coverage does not mitigate racial disparities.[70,119]

Other disparity-targeted interventions have been shown to achieve even greater gains in reducing disparity. One notable example is the C5 initiative executed by the New York City Department of Health and Mental Hygiene, which (1) reduced cost barriers by providing free colonoscopy screening for the uninsured; (2) reduced access barriers by removing the need for specialist consultation before scheduling a screening; and (3) reduced socioeconomic barriers by providing navigators to facilitate transportation and access to affordable medications.[3]

To effectively address disparities present throughout the cancer care continuum (**Fig. 2**), policy changes and interventions must be designed using a multilevel approach. Initiatives should include funding for research to increase enrollment of more diverse populations in clinical trials and to address barriers to treatment beyond simply providing health insurance coverage.[24] Addressing unconscious provider bias is also key. One intervention targeted at providers for patients with lung cancer involved regular individual feedback to providers on treatment completion rates

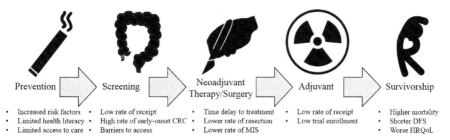

Fig. 2. Disparities along the cancer continuum. DFS, disease-free survival.

among their patients stratified by race as well as real-time warnings on missed care milestones; notably, treatment parity was achieved after implementation.[120]

Finally, there is a growing awareness of the pervasiveness of systemic racism in health care, including but not limited to (1) issues of diversity in the health care workforce and future pipeline, (2) racial bias in the conduct of health research, (3) advances in and reliance on telehealth despite a digital divide, and (4) a lack of diversity curricula and representation in medical education.[121–123] The effects of systemic racism are pervasive and necessitate ongoing vigilant attention and efforts to ensure that all patients have access to equal care.

CLINICS CARE POINTS

- Patients of minority race may not receive adequate treatment for colorectal cancer because of a myriad of barriers including access to care, health insurance, socioeconomic deprivation, patient refusal, and provider bias.

- Advocacy for national, regional, and institution-level interventions to overcome these barriers will be critical to mitigate these treatment disparities.

DISCLOSURE

The authors have nothing to disclose.

REFERENCES

1. Siegel RL, Miller KD, Fuchs HE, et al. Cancer statistics, 2021. CA Cancer J Clin 2021;71(1):7–33.
2. Siegel RL, Miller KD, Sauer AG, et al. Colorectal cancer statistics, 2020. CA Cancer J Clin 2020;70(3):145–64.
3. Polite BN, Gluck AR, Brawley OW. Ensuring equity and justice in the care and outcomes of patients with cancer. JAMA 2019;321(17):1663–4.
4. Popescu I, Schrag D, Ang A, et al. Racial/ethnic and socioeconomic differences in colorectal and breast cancer treatment quality: the role of physician-level variations in care. Med Care 2016;54(8):780–8.
5. Daniel CL, Gilreath K, Keyes D. Colorectal cancer disparities beyond biology: screening, treatment, access. Front Biosci (Landmark Ed) 2017;22:465–78.
6. Lai Y, Wang C, Civan JM, et al. Effects of cancer stage and treatment differences on racial disparities in survival from colon cancer: a united states population-based study. Gastroenterology 2016;150(5):1135–46.
7. Grass F, Behm KT, Duchalais E, et al. Impact of delay to surgery on survival in stage I-III colon cancer. Eur J Surg Oncol 2020;46(3):455–61.
8. Kucejko RJ, Holleran TJ, Stein DE, et al. How soon should patients with colon cancer undergo definitive resection? Dis Colon Rectum 2020;63(2):172–82.
9. Whittaker TM, Abdelrazek MEG, Fitzpatrick AJ, et al. Delay to elective colorectal cancer surgery and implications for survival: a systematic review and meta-analysis. Colorectal Dis 2021. https://doi.org/10.1111/codi.15625.
10. Jones LA, Ferrans CE, Polite BN, et al. Examining racial disparities in colon cancer clinical delay in the colon cancer patterns of care in chicago study. Ann Epidemiol 2017;27(11):731–8.e1.

11. Frankenfeld CL, Menon N, Leslie TF. Racial disparities in colorectal cancer time-to-treatment and survival time in relation to diagnosing hospital cancer-related diagnostic and treatment capabilities. Cancer Epidemiol 2020;65:101684.

12. Eaglehouse YL, Georg MW, Shriver CD, et al. Racial comparisons in timeliness of colon cancer treatment in an equal-access health system. J Natl Cancer Inst 2019;112(4):410–7.

13. Malietzis G, Mughal A, Currie AC, et al. Factors implicated for delay of adjuvant chemotherapy in colorectal cancer: a meta-analysis of observational studies. Ann Surg Oncol 2015;22(12):3793–802.

14. Wasserman DW, Boulos M, Hopman WM, et al. Reasons for delay in time to initiation of adjuvant chemotherapy for colon cancer. J Oncol Pract 2015;11(1):28.

15. Tonlaar N, Song S, Hong JC, et al. Combined-modality therapy for rectal cancer: analysis of potential differences in disease presentation, treatment adherence, and treatment outcome according to race. Am J Clin Oncol 2014;37(2):122–5.

16. Kutikov A, Weinberg DS, Edelman MJ, et al. A war on two fronts: cancer care in the time of COVID-19. Ann Intern Med 2020;172(11):756–8.

17. Larson DW, Abd El Aziz MA, Mandrekar JN. How many lives will delay of colon cancer surgery cost during the COVID-19 pandemic? an analysis based on the US national cancer database. Mayo Clin Proc 2020;95(8):1805–7.

18. Akinyemiju T, Meng Q, Vin-Raviv N. Race/ethnicity and socio-economic differences in colorectal cancer surgery outcomes: analysis of the nationwide inpatient sample. BMC Cancer 2016;16(1):715–7.

19. Bliton JN, Parides M, Muscarella P, et al. Understanding racial disparities in gastrointestinal cancer with mediation analysis: lack of surgery contributes to lower survival in african american patients. Cancer Epidemiol Biomarkers Prev 2021;30(3):529–38.

20. Tramontano AC, Chen Y, Watson TR, et al. Racial/ethnic disparities in colorectal cancer treatment utilization and phase-specific costs, 2000-2014. PloS one 2020;15(4):e0231599.

21. Rodriguez EA, Tamariz L, Palacio A, et al. Racial disparities in the presentation and treatment of colorectal cancer: a statewide cross-sectional study. J Clin Gastroenterol 2018;52(9):817–20.

22. Ellis CT, Samuel CA, Stitzenberg KB. National trends in nonoperative management of rectal adenocarcinoma. J Clin Oncol 2016;34(14):1644–51.

23. Sanford NN, Dee EC, Ahn C, et al. Recent trends and overall survival of young versus older adults with stage II to III rectal cancer treated with and without surgery in the United States, 2010-2015. Am J Clin Oncol 2020;43(10):694–700.

24. American Association for Cancer Research. Philadelphia, PA:AACR cancer disparities progress report 2020 2020. p. 1–145.

25. Fields AC, Lu PW, Yoo J, et al. Treatment of stage I-III rectal cancer: who is refusing surgery? J Surg Oncol 2020;121(6):990–1000.

26. Landrum MB, Keating NL, Lamont EB, et al. Reasons for underuse of recommended therapies for colorectal and lung cancer in the veterans health administration. Cancer 2012;118(13):3345–55.

27. Penner LA, Dovidio JF, Gonzalez R, et al. The effects of oncologist implicit racial bias in racially discordant oncology interactions. J Clin Oncol 2016;34(24):2874–80.

28. Penner LA, Harper FWK, Dovidio JF, et al. The impact of black cancer patients' race-related beliefs and attitudes on racially-discordant oncology interactions: a field study. Soc Sci Med 2017;191:99–108.

29. Baer C, Menon R, Bastawrous S, et al. Emergency presentations of colorectal cancer. Surg Clin North Am 2017;97(3):529–45.

30. Oliphant R, Mansouri D, Nicholson GA, et al. Emergency presentation of node-negative colorectal cancer treated with curative surgery is associated with poorer short and longer-term survival. Int J Colorectal Dis 2014;29(5):591–8.

31. Hogan J, Samaha G, Burke J, et al. Emergency presenting colon cancer is an independent predictor of adverse disease-free survival. Int Surg 2015;100(1):77–86.

32. Wanis KN, Ott M, Van Koughnett J, et al. Long-term oncological outcomes following emergency resection of colon cancer. Int J Colorectal Dis 2018;33(11):1525–32.

33. Moreno CC, Mittal PK, Sullivan PS, et al. Colorectal cancer initial diagnosis: screening colonoscopy, diagnostic colonoscopy, or emergent surgery, and tumor stage and size at initial presentation. Clin Colorectal Cancer 2016;15(1):67–73.

34. Pruitt SL, Davidson NO, Gupta S, et al. Missed opportunities: racial and neighborhood socioeconomic disparities in emergency colorectal cancer diagnosis and surgery. BMC Cancer 2014;14:927.

35. Colon cancer. 2021. Available at: https://www.nccn.org/professionals/physician_gls/pdf/colon.pdf. Accessed April 16, 2021.

36. Gill AA, Zahm SH, Shriver CD, et al. Colon cancer lymph node evaluation among military health system beneficiaries: an analysis by race/ethnicity. Ann Surg Oncol 2015;22(1):195–202.

37. Hsieh MC, Velasco C, Wu XC, et al. Influence of socioeconomic status and hospital type on disparities of lymph node evaluation in colon cancer patients. Cancer 2012;118(6):1675–83.

38. Rhoads KF, Cullen J, Ngo JV, et al. Racial and ethnic differences in lymph node examination after colon cancer resection do not completely explain disparities in mortality. Cancer 2012;118(2):469–77.

39. Hashiguchi Y, Hase K, Ueno H, et al. Impact of race/ethnicity on prognosis in patients who underwent surgery for colon cancer: analysis for white, african, and east asian americans. Ann Surg Oncol 2012;19(5):1517–28.

40. Cone MM, Shoop KM, Rea JD, et al. Ethnicity influences lymph node resection in colon cancer. J Gastrointest Surg 2010;14(11):1752–7.

41. Hall MD, Schultheiss TE, Smith DD, et al. Impact of total lymph node count on staging and survival after neoadjuvant chemoradiation therapy for rectal cancer. Ann Surg Oncol 2015;22(Suppl 3):580.

42. Cheong C, Kim NK. Minimally invasive surgery for rectal cancer: current status and future perspectives. Indian J Surg Oncol 2017;8(4):591–9.

43. Salem JF, Gummadi S, Marks JH. Minimally invasive surgical approaches to colon cancer. Surg Oncol Clin North Am 2018;27(2):303–18.

44. Wells KO, Senagore A. Minimally invasive colon cancer surgery. Surg Oncol Clin North Am 2019;28(2):285–96.

45. Gabriel E, Thirunavukarasu P, Al-Sukhni E, et al. National disparities in minimally invasive surgery for rectal cancer. Surg Endosc 2016;30(3):1060–7.

46. Robinson CN, Balentine CJ, Sansgiry S, et al. Disparities in the use of minimally invasive surgery for colorectal disease. J Gastrointest Surg 2012;16(5):897–903 [discussion: 903–4].

47. Turner M, Adam MA, Sun Z, et al. Insurance status, not race, is associated with use of minimally invasive surgical approach for rectal cancer. Ann Surg 2017;265(4):774–81.

48. Hawkins AT, Ford MM, Benjamin Hopkins M, et al. Barriers to laparoscopic colon resection for cancer: a national analysis. Surg Endosc 2018;32(2):1035–42.

49. Damle RN, Flahive JM, Davids JS, et al. Examination of racial disparities in the receipt of minimally invasive surgery among a national cohort of adult patients undergoing colorectal surgery. Dis Colon Rectum 2016;59(11):1055–62.

50. Osagiede O, Spaulding AC, Cochuyt JJ, et al. Disparities in minimally invasive surgery for colorectal cancer in florida. Am J Surg 2019;218(2):293–301.

51. Bordeianou L, Maguire LH, Alavi K, et al. Sphincter-sparing surgery in patients with low-lying rectal cancer: techniques, oncologic outcomes, and functional results. J Gastrointest Surg 2014;18(7):1358–72.

52. Paquette IM, Kemp JA, Finlayson SR. Patient and hospital factors associated with use of sphincter-sparing surgery for rectal cancer. Dis Colon Rectum 2010;53(2):115–20.

53. Arsoniadis EG, Fan Y, Jarosek S, et al. Decreased use of sphincter-preserving procedures among african americans with rectal cancer. Ann Surg Oncol 2018;25(3):720–8.

54. Cairns AL, Schlottmann F, Strassle PD, et al. Racial and socioeconomic disparities in the surgical management and outcomes of patients with colorectal carcinoma. World J Surg 2019;43(5):1342–50.

55. Chan SY, Suwanabol PA, Damle RN, et al. Characterizing short-term outcomes following surgery for rectal cancer: the role of race and insurance status. J Gastrointest Surg 2016;20(11):1891–8.

56. Sharp SP, Ata A, Chismark AD, et al. Racial disparities after stoma construction in colorectal surgery. Colorectal Dis 2020;22(6):713–22.

57. Leeds IL, Alimi Y, Hobson DR, et al. Racial and socioeconomic differences manifest in process measure adherence for enhanced recovery after surgery pathway. Dis Colon Rectum 2017;60(10):1092–101.

58. Wahl TS, Goss LE, Morris MS, et al. Enhanced recovery after surgery (ERAS) eliminates racial disparities in postoperative length of stay after colorectal surgery. Ann Surg 2018;268(6):1026–35.

59. Feeney G, Sehgal R, Sheehan M, et al. Neoadjuvant radiotherapy for rectal cancer management. World J Gastroenterol 2019;25(33):4850–69.

60. São Julião GP, Habr-Gama A, Vailati BB, et al. New strategies in rectal cancer. Surg Clin North Am 2017;97(3):587–604.

61. Rectal cancer. 2020. Available at: https://www.nccn.org/professionals/physician_gls/pdf/rectal.pdf. Accessed April 16, 2021.

62. Ofshteyn A, Bingmer K, Dorth J, et al. Disparities in neoadjuvant radiation dosing for treatment of rectal cancer. Am J Surg 2020;220(4):987–92.

63. Sineshaw HM, Jemal A, Thomas CR Jr, et al. Changes in treatment patterns for patients with locally advanced rectal cancer in the united states over the past decade: an analysis from the national cancer data base. Cancer 2016;122(13):1996–2003.

64. Wong DL, Hendrick LE, Guerrero WM, et al. Adherence to neoadjuvant therapy guidelines for locally advanced rectal cancers in a region with sociodemographic disparities. Am J Surg 2020. https://doi.org/10.1016/j.amjsurg.2020.11.049.

65. McClure LA, Sussman DA, Hernandez MN, et al. Factors associated with receipt of radiation therapy for rectal cancer. Am J Clin Oncol 2018;41(3):227–9.

66. Bender U, Rho YS, Barrera I, et al. Adjuvant therapy for stages II and III colon cancer: risk stratification, treatment duration, and future directions. Curr Oncol 2019;26(Suppl 1):S43–52.

67. Moertel CG, Fleming TR, Macdonald JS, et al. Intergroup study of fluorouracil plus levamisole as adjuvant therapy for stage II/dukes' B2 colon cancer. J Clin Oncol 1995;13(12):2936–43.

68. André T, Boni C, Mounedji-Boudiaf L, et al. Oxaliplatin, fluorouracil, and leucovorin as adjuvant treatment for colon cancer. N Engl J Med 2004;350(23): 2343–51.

69. Schmoll HJ, Tabernero J, Maroun J, et al. Capecitabine plus oxaliplatin compared with fluorouracil/folinic acid as adjuvant therapy for stage III colon cancer: final results of the NO16968 randomized controlled phase III trial. J Clin Oncol 2015;33(32):3733–40.

70. Murphy CC, Harlan LC, Warren JL, et al. Race and insurance differences in the receipt of adjuvant chemotherapy among patients with stage III colon cancer. J Clin Oncol 2015;33(23):2530–6.

71. Gorey KM, Haji-Jama S, Bartfay E, et al. Lack of access to chemotherapy for colon cancer: multiplicative disadvantage of being extremely poor, inadequately insured and african american. BMC Health Serv Res 2014;14:133.

72. Becerra AZ, Probst CP, Tejani MA, et al. Opportunity lost: adjuvant chemotherapy in patients with stage III colon cancer remains underused. Surgery 2015;158(3):692–9.

73. Hsieh MC, Chiu YW, Velasco C, et al. Impact of race/ethnicity and socioeconomic status on adjuvant chemotherapy use among elderly patients with stage III colon cancer. J Registry Manag 2013;40(4):180–7.

74. Hu CY, Delclos GL, Chan W, et al. Assessing the initiation and completion of adjuvant chemotherapy in a large nationwide and population-based cohort of elderly patients with stage-III colon cancer. Med Oncol 2011;28(4):1062–74.

75. Turner MC, Farrow NE, Rhodin KE, et al. Delay in adjuvant chemotherapy and survival advantage in stage III colon cancer. J Am Coll Surg 2018;226(4):670–8.

76. Upadhyay S, Dahal S, Bhatt VR, et al. Chemotherapy use in stage III colon cancer: a national cancer database analysis. Ther Adv Med Oncol 2015;7(5): 244–51.

77. Sinicrope FA, Ou F, Nixon AB, et al. Randomized trial of standard chemotherapy alone or combined with atezolizumab as adjuvant therapy for patients with stage III colon cancer and deficient mismatch repair (ATOMIC, alliance A021502). J Clin Oncol 2019;37(15):e15169.

78. Cheong CK, Nistala KRY, Ng CH, et al. Neoadjuvant therapy in locally advanced colon cancer: a meta-analysis and systematic review. J Gastrointest Oncol 2020;11(5):847–57.

79. Willett CG. Management of locoregional rectal cancer. J Natl Compr Canc Netw 2018;16(5S):617–9.

80. Lu PW, Scully RE, Fields AC, et al. Racial disparities in treatment for rectal cancer at minority-serving hospitals. J Gastrointest Surg 2020. https://doi.org/10. 1007/s11605-020-04744-x.

81. Xu Z, Mohile SG, Tejani MA, et al. Poor compliance with adjuvant chemotherapy use associated with poorer survival in patients with rectal cancer: an NCDB analysis. Cancer 2017;123(1):52–61.

82. Daly MC, Jung AD, Hanseman DJ, et al. Surviving rectal cancer: examination of racial disparities surrounding access to care. J Surg Res 2017;211:100–6.

83. Quinn TJ, Rajagopalan MS, Gill B, et al. Patterns of care and outcomes for adjuvant treatment of pT3N0 rectal cancer using the national cancer database. J Gastrointest Oncol 2020;11(1):1–12.

84. Pulte D, Jansen L, Brenner H. Social disparities in survival after diagnosis with colorectal cancer: Contribution of race and insurance status. Cancer Epidemiol 2017;48:41–7.

85. Ghaffarpasand E, Welten VM, Fields AC, et al. Racial and socioeconomic disparities after surgical resection for rectal cancer. J Surg Res 2020;256:449–57.

86. Tawk R, Abner A, Ashford A, et al. Differences in colorectal cancer outcomes by race and insurance. Int J Environ Res Public Health 2015;13(1):48.

87. Cabo J, Shu X, Shu XO, et al. Treatment at academic centers decreases insurance-based survival disparities in colon cancer. J Surg Res 2020;245: 265–72.

88. Snyder RA, Hu CY, Zafar SN, et al. Racial disparities in recurrence and overall survival in patients with locoregional colorectal cancer. J Natl Cancer Inst 2020. https://doi.org/10.1093/jnci/djaa182.

89. Dignam JJ, Ye Y, Colangelo L, et al. Prognosis after rectal cancer in blacks and whites participating in adjuvant therapy randomized trials. J Clin Oncol 2003; 21(3):413–20.

90. Yoon HH, Shi Q, Alberts SR, et al. Racial differences in BRAF/KRAS mutation rates and survival in stage III colon cancer patients. J Natl Cancer Inst 2015; 107(10):djv186.

91. Yothers G, Sargent DJ, Wolmark N, et al. Outcomes among black patients with stage II and III colon cancer receiving chemotherapy: an analysis of ACCENT adjuvant trials. J Natl Cancer Inst 2011;103(20):1498–506.

92. Hines RB, Jiban MJH, Lee E, et al. Characteristics associated with nonreceipt of surveillance testing and the relationship with survival in stage II and III colon cancer. Am J Epidemiol 2020;190(2):239–50.

93. Howlader N, Noone AM, Krapcho M, et al, editors. SEER cancer statistics review, 1975-2018. Bethesda, MD: National Cancer Institute; 2021. Available at: https://seer.cancer.gov/csr/1975_2018/. Accessed April 24, 2021.

94. Frick MA, Vachani CC, Hampshire MK, et al. Survivorship after lower gastrointestinal cancer: patient-reported outcomes and planning for care. Cancer 2017;123(10):1860–8.

95. Belachew AA, Reyes ME, Ye Y, et al. Patterns of racial/ethnic disparities in baseline health-related quality of life and relationship with overall survival in patients with colorectal cancer. Qual Life Res 2020;29(11):2977–86.

96. Rao D, Debb S, Blitz D, et al. Racial/ethnic differences in the health-related quality of life of cancer patients. J Pain Symptom Manage 2008;36(5):488–96.

97. Hastert TA, Kyko JM, Reed AR, et al. Financial hardship and quality of life among african american and white cancer survivors: the role of limiting care due to cost. Cancer Epidemiol Biomarkers Prev 2019;28(7):1202–11.

98. Hastert TA, McDougall JA, Strayhorn SM, et al. Social needs and health-related quality of life among african american cancer survivors: results from the detroit research on cancer survivors study. Cancer 2020. https://doi.org/10.1002/cncr.33286.

99. Al-Husseini MJ, Saad AM, Jazieh KA, et al. Outcome disparities in colorectal cancer: a SEER-based comparative analysis of racial subgroups. Int J Colorectal Dis 2019;34(2):285–92.

100. Javid SH, Varghese TK, Morris AM, et al. Guideline-concordant cancer care and survival among american indian/alaskan native patients. Cancer 2014;120(14): 2183–90.

101. Cueto CV, Szeja S, Wertheim BC, et al. Disparities in treatment and survival of white and native american patients with colorectal cancer: a SEER analysis. J Am Coll Surg 2011;213(4):469–74.
102. Mulhern KC, Wahl TS, Goss LE, et al. Reduced disparities and improved surgical outcomes for asian americans with colorectal cancer. J Surg Res 2017; 218:23–8.
103. Mauri G, Sartore-Bianchi A, Russo AG, et al. Early-onset colorectal cancer in young individuals. Mol Oncol 2019;13(2):109–31.
104. Murphy CC, Wallace K, Sandler RS, et al. Racial disparities in incidence of young-onset colorectal cancer and patient survival. Gastroenterology 2019; 156(4):958–65.
105. Koblinski J, Jandova J, Nfonsam V. Disparities in incidence of early- and late-onset colorectal cancer between hispanics and whites: a 10-year SEER database study. Am J Surg 2018;215(4):581–5.
106. Crosbie AB, Roche LM, Johnson LM, et al. Trends in colorectal cancer incidence among younger adults-disparities by age, sex, race, ethnicity, and subsite. Cancer Med 2018;7(8):4077–86.
107. Wu J, Ye J, Wu W, et al. Racial disparities in young-onset patients with colorectal, breast and testicular cancer. J Cancer 2019;10(22):5388–96.
108. Ewongwo A, Hamidi M, Alattar Z, et al. Contributing factors and short-term surgical outcomes of patients with early-onset rectal cancer. Am J Surg 2020; 219(4):578–82.
109. Lee DY, Teng A, Pedersen RC, et al. Racial and socioeconomic treatment disparities in adolescents and young adults with stage II-III rectal cancer. Ann Surg Oncol 2017;24(2):311–8.
110. Alese OB, Jiang R, Zakka KM, et al. Analysis of racial disparities in the treatment and outcomes of colorectal cancer in young adults. Cancer Epidemiol 2019;63: 101618.
111. Quinn TJ, Kabolizadeh P. Rectal cancer in young patients: Incidence and outcome disparities. J Gastrointest Oncol 2020;11(5):880–93.
112. Dharwadkar P, Greenan G, Stoffel EM, et al. Racial and ethnic disparities in germline genetic testing of patients with young-onset colorectal cancer. Clin Gastroenterol Hepatol 2020. https://doi.org/10.1016/j.cgh.2020.12.025.
113. American cancer society guideline for colorectal cancer screening. Available at: https://www.cancer.org/cancer/colon-rectal-cancer/detection-diagnosis-staging/acs-recommendations.html. Accessed April 17, 2021.
114. Ellis L, Canchola AJ, Spiegel D, et al. Racial and ethnic disparities in cancer survival: the contribution of tumor, sociodemographic, institutional, and neighborhood characteristics. J Clin Oncol 2018;36(1):25–33.
115. Dumenci L, Matsuyama R, Riddle DL, et al. Measurement of cancer health literacy and identification of patients with limited cancer health literacy. J Health Commun 2014;19(Suppl 2):205–24.
116. Snyder RA, Chang GJ. Insurance status as a surrogate for social determinants of health in cancer clinical trials. JAMA Netw Open 2020;3(4):e203890.
117. Sabik LM, Adunlin G. The ACA and cancer screening and diagnosis. Cancer J 2017;23(3):151–62.
118. Loehrer AP, Song Z, Haynes AB, et al. Impact of health insurance expansion on the treatment of colorectal cancer. J Clin Oncol 2016;34(34):4110–5.
119. Hao S, Snyder R, Irish W, et al. Explaining disparities in colon cancer treatment: differential effects of health insurance by race. J Am Coll Surg 2020;231(4): S55–6.

120. Cykert S, Eng E, Walker P, et al. A system-based intervention to reduce black-white disparities in the treatment of early stage lung cancer: a pragmatic trial at five cancer centers. Cancer Med 2019;8(3):1095–102.

121. Evans MK, Rosenbaum L, Malina D, et al. Diagnosing and treating systemic racism. N Engl J Med 2020;383(3):274–6.

122. Newman LA. Cascading consequences of systemic racism on public health. Ann Surg 2021;273(1):10–2.

123. Rodriguez JA, Clark CR, Bates DW. Digital health equity as a necessity in the 21st century cures act era. JAMA 2020;323(23):2381–2.

Breast Cancer Disparities and the Impact of Geography

Samilia Obeng-Gyasi, MD, MPH[a],*, Barnabas Obeng-Gyasi, BS[b],
Willi Tarver, DrPH, MLIS[c]

KEYWORDS

- Rural • Urban • Neighborhood • Breast cancer • Disparities

KEY POINTS

- Neighborhood is a powerful social determinant of health with significant implications for breast cancer outcomes.
- High neighborhood deprivation is associated with advanced stages of disease at presentation and disparities in locoregional and systemic treatment.
- Rural patients with breast cancer face barriers in screening and treatment of breast cancer that adversely affect their survival.

INTRODUCTION

National discussions of health disparities and health equity have placed a spotlight on social determinants of health (SDH). SDHs describe living and working conditions that affect overall health and influence one's ability to achieve health equity.[1,2] In the United States, place of residence has emerged as a powerful SDH, with some scholars suggesting that zip code is more significant for health outcomes than genetic code.[3] This assertion is rooted in the effects of governmental policy, societal values, and cultural norms on the creation of neighborhoods and its subsequent implications for health and health outcomes.[2] For example, in the 1930s, systemic racism informed the practice of redlining by the Federal Housing Administration and the Home Owners' Loan Corporation.[4,5] Redlining is the practice of systematic residential segregation by race in conjunction with disinvestment in Black neighborhoods secondary to mortgage lending biases.[4] This historical practice has resulted in pervasive and persistent

[a] Division of Surgical Oncology, Department of Surgery, The Ohio State University, N924 Doan Hall, 410 West 10th, Columbus, OH 43210, USA; [b] Department of Radiology, Duke University Medical Center, 10 Duke Medicine Circle, Durham, NC 27710, USA; [c] Division of Cancer Prevention & Control, Department of Internal Medicine, College of Medicine, The Ohio State University, 460 Medical Center Drive, Room 526, Columbus, OH 43210, USA
* Corresponding author.
E-mail address: samilia.obeng-gyasi@osumc.edu
Twitter: @GyasiSamilia (S.O.-G.)

Surg Oncol Clin N Am 31 (2022) 81–90
https://doi.org/10.1016/j.soc.2021.08.002
1055-3207/22/© 2021 Elsevier Inc. All rights reserved.

surgonc.theclinics.com

inequities and inequalities between predominantly Black versus White neighbor-hoods.[5] Moreover, it has also adversely affected other SDHs such as education, employment, and homeownership in Black communities.[5]

The terms neighborhood, place, and area of residence all describe where people live. Neighborhood as a SDH can be viewed through its components of the built environment, services, and the people within the neighborhood.[6] The built environment describes the infrastructure of a neighborhood such as buildings, streets, parks, and playgrounds.[7] Examples of how the built environment can influence health outcomes include higher rates of obesity in neighborhoods with poor walkability.[8] Services within a neighborhood include employment opportunities, schools, housing, and access to hospitals.[6] Social relationships describe interactions between community members and how they leverage social cohesion and social capital within those relationships.[9] These multidimensional components of the neighborhood influence health behaviors and psychosocial stressors and can even result in epigenetic changes (**Fig. 1**).[6,10]

Social epigenetics is an emerging field evaluating the impact of the social and built environment on transcription of genetic information.[6] Specifically, current research suggests epigenetic changes secondary to the social and built environment result in alterations in RNA silencing, protein folding, DNA methylation, and histone modification.[6] These epigenetic changes provide a plausible mechanism for how environmental exposures and chronic socioeconomic deprivation alter DNA and subsequently promote disease initiation and progression.[6] For instance, epigenetic changes have been implicated in racial disparities in squamous cell carcinoma of the head and neck, depressive symptoms, and the development of hormone receptor-negative breast cancers among Black women.[11–13]

The impact of place across the cancer continuum from prevention through survivorship is an area of active research. For patients with breast cancer in particular, current studies suggest area of residence is a determinant of breast cancer stage of diagnosis, treatment, and mortality.[14,15] The objective of this article is to provide a contemporary overview of the impact of place of residence on screening, stage, treatment, and mortality among patients with breast cancer. Place will be examined through the lens of neighborhood and rural–urban status.

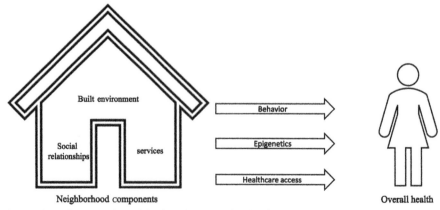

Fig. 1. The influence of neighborhood on health. This figure depicts the pathways through which neighborhood can influence health.

DISCUSSION
Neighborhood and Breast Cancer Screening, Stage, Treatment, and Mortality

Screening and stage at diagnosis

The Healthy People 2030 target for breast cancer screening among US women is 77.1% of women ages 50 to 74.[16] However, current estimates project that approximately 72.8% of women within that age range undergo screening.[17] Factors affecting screening rates involve a combination of patient-related (eg, cultural beliefs) and structural variables, such as the availability of screening mammography facilities.[18,19] Neighborhood, as a determinant of health, influences screening rates by either mitigating or creating barriers in health care access, quality, and timeliness of care.

Neighborhood characteristics associated with a lower adherence to breast cancer screening guidelines include living in the inner city, rurality, high neighborhood socioeconomic deprivation, and no primary care facilities within a neighborhood.[20,21] Of note, patients living in neighborhoods with greater socioeconomic deprivation face longer times to diagnostic resolution after an abnormal mammogram compared with those in areas with low deprivation.[22] In Beyer and colleagues' evaluation of perceived neighborhood quality and screening among Wisconsin residents, low levels of neighborhood stress were associated with an increased odds of undergoing screening mammography.[23]

Neighborhood-based disparities in screening could have significant repercussions for stage at diagnosis, breast cancer tumor subtype, and mortality. A recent evaluation of patients with nonmetastatic breast cancer in the Surveillance Epidemiology and End Results database showed patients living in neighborhoods with low socioeconomic status were more likely to present with stage III breast cancer compared with their counterparts in more affluent neighborhoods.[24] Moreover, Black women are more likely to live in neighborhoods characterized by higher levels of socioeconomic disadvantage, and Black people are more likely to present with triple-negative breast cancer, an aggressive breast cancer subtype.[25] However, studies evaluating the relationship between neighborhood racial segregation and breast cancer stage suggest racial segregation may not influence breast cancer stage.[26]

Treatment

Locoregional management: Surgery and radiation therapy. A recent examination of neighborhood characteristics and locoregional management in the Missouri state registry revealed that patients living in neighborhoods with greater deprivation were more likely to undergo mastectomy or have surgical management omitted altogether. Additionally, those in areas with greater deprivation had no or delayed radiation therapy after breast-conserving surgery.[27] Among adolescent and young adult patients with breast cancer (defined as ages 15–39) increased mastectomy use, as well as omission of radiation therapy after breast-conserving surgery are associated with residency in neighborhoods with low socioeconomic status.[28]

Wakefield and colleagues[29] conducted a study of radiation therapy interruptions in a cohort of patients with cancer that included patients with breast cancer. Their results suggest residing in a low-income neighborhood increased the likelihood of 5 or more unplanned radiation therapy appointment cancellations.[29]

Unfortunately, there are very few contemporary studies evaluating the relationship between locoregional management and neighborhood. Consequently, there are gaps in the literature on the relationship between neighborhood and receipt of contralateral prophylactic mastectomy (CPM) or breast reconstruction. Moreover, the influence of neighborhood on adherence to omitting low-value surgical procedures such as lymph node surgery in women aged 70 years or greater with small hormone receptor-positive breast cancers warrants investigation.[30]

Systemic treatment. Significant advances have been made over the past half century on systemic therapies for breast cancer. With the advent of novel chemotherapeutic agents, endocrine therapy, and targeted therapies for the human epidermal growth factor receptor (HER2/neu), breast cancer management has transitioned from mostly local therapies to a combination of local and systemic treatments.[31,32] Regrettably, there is a dearth of literature on the effects of neighborhood on receipt of systemic therapies. Sadigh and colleagues[33] reviewed the Trial Assigning Individualized Options for Treatment (Rx) (TAILORx trial) and showed an association between high neighborhood deprivation and early discontinuation of endocrine therapy. The study findings are noteworthy because they suggested that, after controlling for neighborhood deprivation, Black patients with breast cancer in the trial had higher rates of adherence to hormone therapy than White women. The TAILORx trial evaluated the benefit of chemotherapy among hormone receptor-positive, HER2/neu-negative patients with breast cancer stratified by the Oncotype Dx Recurrence score.[34]

Mortality

Residing in neighborhoods with low socioeconomic status or high rates of deprivation is associated with greater mortality among patients with breast cancer.[35,36] To determine the association between neighborhood and survival, Shariff-Marco and colleagues[37] aggregated neighborhoods based on demographics and household composition, immigration, neighborhood socioeconomic status, walkability, residential mobility, commuting, rural/urban status, land use, and food environment to create neighborhood archetypes. The study results suggest that overall and breast cancer-specific survival are associated with neighborhood archetype. Specifically, patients in upper middle class neighborhoods with a high socioeconomic status had the highest survival rates.[37]

The legacy of redlining has been implicated in increasing breast cancer mortality.[38] In a study by Collin and colleagues,[38] both Black and White patients living in areas of high redlining had higher mortality compared with patients living in areas of low redlining. Conversely, residency in a neighborhood with lending bias, defined as race-based systematic denial of mortgages, was associated with decreased breast cancer mortality.[38] Interestingly, for Black women, residing in neighborhoods with increasing proportions of Black people was associated with lower morality.[26] These findings are in contrast with Russel and colleagues'[39] work showing higher mortality rates among Black women in neighborhoods with higher percentages of Black residents.

Impact of Rural–Urban Status on Breast Cancer Screening, Treatment, and Mortality

Screening and stage

Studies evaluating the relationship between rural–urban status and mammography use have been inconsistent about the effects of rurality on receipt of mammography. Examinations of both national and state databases suggest rural women are less likely to undergo screening mammography compared with women living in urban areas.[40–42] This pattern of care is also prevalent among sexual minorities, with rural women who identify as lesbians having lower screening rates than urban heterosexual women.[43] Explanations for disparities in screening rates include lower access and longer driving times to screening facilities.[40,44,45] Conversely, Henry and colleagues'[46] review of Utah's Behavioral Risk Factor Surveillance System did not show a statistically significant association between geographic factors and mammography use. Moreover, a review of mammography receipt at the national, regional, and state levels using the Behavioral Risk Factor Surveillance System only showed small differences between women living in rural versus urban areas.[47]

The inconsistency across study results of the implications of rurality on screening are interesting within the context of the study by Davis and colleagues[48] examining and comparing barriers, knowledge, and experiences between rural and urban women receiving care at federally qualified health centers in Louisiana. In this study, rural women, despite having low knowledge about when to initiate screening, had positive beliefs and fewer barriers to undergoing mammography than women living in urban areas. Specifically, rural women were more likely to report a physician recommendation for mammography, less likely to find mammography embarrassing, and seemed to be less afraid of possibly receiving a positive result.[48]

These discrepancies in the association between rural–urban status and screening require further investigation as screening mammography is associated with a reduction in breast cancer-specific mortality.[49] And despite the aforementioned behavioral and psychological characteristics among rural women vis a vis breast cancer screening, studies indicate rural patients with breast cancer present with more advanced stages of breast cancer, which could be the result of additional, unmeasured barriers to screening.[50,51] It is anticipated that differences in the discussed study results are most likely secondary to differences in study timeframes and the contribution of other SDH (eg, insurance).

Treatment
Locoregional management: Surgery and radiation therapy. Surgical management is an important component of the multidisciplinary care of breast cancer, with the majority of patients with stages I to III disease undergoing surgery.[52] A recent study evaluating surgical management across the rural-urban continuum in the National Cancer Database (NCDB) showed there was no difference in the use of mastectomy between patients based on area of residence.[53] However, Longacre and colleagues[54] evaluation of the Surveillance Epidemiology and End Result program suggests patients living more than 50 miles from a radiation facility are more likely to undergo mastectomy compared with patients living closer to a facility. The discrepancy in results between the NCDB and Surveillance Epidemiology and End Results is mostly likely a reflection of the sociodemographic profiles of the populations in both datasets. Additionally, patients in the NCDB are receiving treatment in Commission on Cancer hospitals, which have specific accreditation requirements that could be influencing treatment decisions.

Although breast reconstruction use among postmastectomy rural patients seems to be increasing, rates still lag behind those of patients living in large metropolitan areas.[53,55] In Obeng-Gyasi and colleagues'[53] review of reconstructive surgery use among post-mastectomy patients, individuals living in large metropolitan areas had a 25% increased odds of undergoing reconstruction compared with those in rural areas. A possible driver of rural–urban disparities in reconstruction is the geographic availability of reconstructive surgeons.[56]

Currently, the American Society of Breast Surgeons, the Society of Surgical Oncology, and Choosing Wisely guidelines discourage women with unilateral cancers without underlying genetic mutations from undergoing CPM.[30] Nevertheless, there has been a significant increase in the use of CPM with young women as the main drivers of this trend.[57] This pattern of young age and increased CPM use has also been seen among rural patients. In an examination of CPM among patients with breast cancer in Iowa, young (defined as aged <40 years), rural women had the highest rate of CPM compared with metropolitan and nonmetropolitan women. Notably, in the aforementioned study, rural women who traveled to metropolitan hospitals had higher rates of CPM than those who were treated at rural hospitals.[58]

Locoregional management of breast cancer with breast conservation surgery in conjunction with radiation (ie, breast conservation therapy) is effective in reducing recurrence.[59] The receipt of radiation therapy after breast conservation therapy in patients with early stage breast cancer is considered guideline-concordant care.[54] Studies indicate the main barrier to use of radiation therapy among rural patients are long travel distances.[54]

Systemic treatment. Unfortunately, there is a paucity of literature on the relationship between rural-urban status and systemic treatments. In Andreason and colleagues'[60] retrospective multi-institutional review, there was no difference in the use of hormone therapy based on rural versus urban residency. However, when stratified by Oncotype Dx recurrence score, rural patients with a recurrence score of 18 to 30 were less likely to undergo chemotherapy than urban patients with a similar score.[60] With the results of the recent RxPONDER trial (examining benefit of chemotherapy in women with hormone receptor-positive, HER2-negative disease, 1–3 positive lymph nodes, and low-risk recurrence score) and the aforementioned TAILORx trial, additional studies are needed to evaluate the dissemination and implementation of these trial results on systemic therapies in hormone receptor–positive patients across the rural–urban continuum.

Mortality. National mortality rates from cancer seem to be on the decline.[61] However, rural patients may not be experiencing decreases in mortality rates comparable with their urban counterparts.[61] In patients with breast cancer, the relationship between rural–urban status and mortality is unclear. Chu and colleagues'[62] review of the Louisiana Tumor Registry suggest differences in overall and disease-specific survival among rural and urban patients with breast cancer are driven by sociodemographic, clinical, and treatment variables rather than area of residence. Conversely, an examination of the NCDB showed patients with breast cancer living in large metropolitan areas have an 8% relative risk reduction in overall mortality compared with patients living in rural areas after controlling for sociodemographic, clinical, and treatment factors.[53] The inconsistency in these results may be reflective of the patient populations used in each study. The NCDB represents approximately 70% of cancers in the United States and consequently may have a more heterogeneous population compared with the registry of the state of Louisiana.[62]

SUMMARY

Area of residence has significant implications for breast cancer screening, stage of diagnosis, treatment, and mortality. However, there are significant gaps in the literature on the impact of neighborhood on the receipt or completion of systemic therapies. Moreover, additional research needs to be conducted on how place influences emerging changes in surgical management such as implementation of axillary surgery de-escalation, elimination of low-value surgical procedures, and the use of oncoplastic reconstruction. Health systems need to incorporate population health into their healthcare delivery paradigms to help identify and address the effects of place on breast cancer outcomes.

CLINICS CARE POINTS

- Routinely collect SDH as part of clinic workflow to identify barriers faced by patients in rural or high deprivation neighborhoods.
- Incorporate social work or patient navigation to help mitigate barriers.

DISCLOSURE

S. Obeng-Gyasi is funded by the Paul Calabresi Career Development Award (K12 CA133250). B. Obeng-Gyasi and W. Tarver have nothing to disclose.

REFERENCES

1. Artiga Samantha HE. Beyond Health Care: The Role of Social Determinants in Promoting Health and Health Equity. Kaiser Family Foundation; 2018. Available at: https://www.kff.org/disparities-policy/issue-brief/beyond-health-care-the-role-of-social-determinants-in-promoting-health-and-health-equity/. Accessed September 15, 2019.
2. Solar O, Irwin A. A conceptual framework for action on the social determinants of health. Social Determinants of Health Discussion Paper 2 (Policy and Practice). 2010. Accessed March 11, 2020. Available at: https://www.who.int/sdhconference/resources/ConceptualframeworkforactiononSDH_eng.pdf.
3. Graham GN. Why your ZIP code matters more than your genetic code: promoting healthy outcomes from mother to child. Breastfeed Med 2016;11:396–7.
4. Fritz M. Federal Housing Administration (FHA). Encyclopedia Britannica. August 9, 2019. 2021. Available at: https://www.britannica.com/topic/Federal-Housing-Administration. Accessed April 24, 2021.
5. Richardson B. Redlining's legacy of inequality: low homeownership rates, less equity for Black households. Forbes. 2020. Available at: https://www.forbes.com/sites/brendarichardson/2020/06/11/redlinings-legacy-of-inequality-low-homeownership-rates-less-equity-for-black-households/?sh=2d4acfc12a7c. Accessed April 24, 2021.
6. Bharmal N, Derose KP, Felician MF, et al. Understanding the Upstream social determinants of health. RAND Corporation; 2015. Available at: https://www.rand.org/pubs/working_papers/WR1096.html.
7. Perdue WC, Stone LA, Gostin LO. The built environment and its relationship to the public's health: the legal framework. Am J Public Health 2003;93(9):1390–4.
8. Kowaleski-Jones L, Zick C, Smith KR, et al. Walkable neighborhoods and obesity: evaluating effects with a propensity score approach. SSM Popul Health 2018;6:9–15.
9. Gomez SL, Shariff-Marco S, DeRouen M, et al. The impact of neighborhood social and built environment factors across the cancer continuum: current research, methodological considerations, and future directions. Cancer 2015;121(14):2314–30.
10. Evans L, Engelman M, Mikulas A, et al. How are social determinants of health integrated into epigenetic research? A systematic review. Social Sci Med (1982) 2021;273:113738.
11. Ambrosone CB, Young AC, Sucheston LE, et al. Genome-wide methylation patterns provide insight into differences in breast tumor biology between American women of African and European ancestry. Oncotarget 2014;5(1):237–48.
12. Lei MK, Beach SR, Simons RL, et al. Neighborhood crime and depressive symptoms among African American women: genetic moderation and epigenetic mediation of effects. Social Sci Med (1982) 2015;146:120–8.
13. Guerrero-Preston R, Lawson F, Rodriguez-Torres S, et al. JAK3 variant, immune signatures, DNA methylation, and social determinants linked to survival racial disparities in head and neck cancer patients. Cancer Prev Res (Phila) 2019;12(4):255–70.

14. Obeng-Gyasi S, Timsina L, Miller KD, et al. The implications of insurance status on presentation, surgical management, and mortality among nonmetastatic breast cancer patients in Indiana. Surgery 2018;164(6):1366–71.

15. John Kollman HL, Sobotka. Poverty and cancer disparities in Ohio 2019. Available at: https://www.cdc.gov/pcd/issues/2018/18_0332.htm. Accessed April 25, 2019.

16. Office of Disease Prevention and Health Promotion OotASfH, Office of the Secretary, U.S. Department of Health and Human Services. . Increase the proportion of females who get screened for breast cancer — C-05. 2021. Available at: https://health.gov/healthypeople/objectives-and-data/browse-objectives/cancer/increase-proportion-females-who-get-screened-breast-cancer-c-05. Accessed April 27, 2021.

17. Sabatino SA, Thompson TD, White MC, et al. Cancer screening test receipt — United States. MMWR Morb Mortal Wkly Rep 2021;2018(70):29–35.

18. Elkin EB, Ishill NM, Snow JG, et al. Geographic access and the use of screening mammography. Med Care 2010;48(4):349–56.

19. Russell KM, Monahan P, Wagle A, et al. Differences in health and cultural beliefs by stage of mammography screening adoption in African American women. Cancer 2007;109(2 Suppl):386–95.

20. Kurani SS, McCoy RG, Lampman MA, et al. Association of neighborhood measures of social determinants of health with breast, cervical, and colorectal cancer screening rates in the US Midwest. JAMA Netw Open 2020;3(3):e200618.

21. Millon-Underwood S, Kelber ST. Exploratory study of breast cancer screening practices of urban women: a closer look at who is and is not getting screened. ABNF J 2015;26(2):30–8.

22. Plascak JJ, Llanos AA, Pennell ML, et al. Neighborhood factors associated with time to resolution following an abnormal breast or cervical cancer screening test. Cancer Epidemiol Biomarkers Prev 2014;23(12):2819–28.

23. Beyer KM, Malecki KM, Hoormann KA, et al. Perceived neighborhood quality and cancer screening behavior: evidence from the Survey of the Health of Wisconsin. J Community Health 2016;41(1):134–7.

24. Abdel-Rahman O. Impact of NCI Socioeconomic Index on the outcomes of non-metastatic breast cancer patients: analysis of SEER census tract-level socioeconomic database. Clin Breast Cancer 2019;19(6):e717–22.

25. Qin B, Babel RA, Plascak JJ, et al. Neighborhood social environmental factors and breast cancer subtypes among Black women. Cancer Epidemiol biomarkers Prev 2021;30(2):344–50.

26. Warner ET, Gomez SL. Impact of neighborhood racial composition and metropolitan residential segregation on disparities in breast cancer stage at diagnosis and survival between black and white women in California. J Community Health 2010;35(4):398–408.

27. Zhang S, Liu Y, Yun S, et al. Impacts of neighborhood characteristics on treatment and outcomes in women with ductal carcinoma in situ of the breast. Cancer Epidemiol biomarkers Prev 2018;27(11):1298–306.

28. Derouen MC, Gomez SL, Press DJ, et al. A population-based observational study of first-course treatment and survival for adolescent and young adult females with breast cancer. J Adolesc Young Adult Oncol 2013;2(3):95–103.

29. Wakefield DV, Carnell M, Dove APH, et al. Location as destiny: identifying geospatial disparities in radiation treatment interruption by neighborhood, race, and insurance. Int J Radiat Oncol Biol Phys 2020;107(4):815–26.

30. Wang T, Baskin AS, Dossett LA. Deimplementation of the Choosing Wisely recommendations for low-value breast cancer surgery: a systematic review. JAMA Surg 2020. https://doi.org/10.1001/jamasurg.2020.0322.
31. Mamounas EP. NSABP breast cancer clinical trials: recent results and future directions. Clin Med Res 2003;1(4):309–26.
32. Slamon D, Eiermann W, Robert N, et al. Adjuvant trastuzumab in HER2-positive breast cancer. N Engl J Med 2011;365(14):1273–83.
33. Sadigh G, Gray RJ, Sparano JA, et al. Breast cancer patients' insurance status and residence zip code correlate with early discontinuation of endocrine therapy: an analysis of the ECOG-ACRIN TAILORx trial. Cancer 2021. https://doi.org/10.1002/cncr.33527.
34. Sparano JA, Gray RJ, Makower DF, et al. Adjuvant chemotherapy guided by a 21-gene expression assay in breast cancer. N Engl J Med 2018;379(2):111–21.
35. O'Brien B, Koru-Sengul T, Miao F, et al. Disparities in overall survival for male breast cancer patients in the state of Florida (1996-2007). Clin Breast Cancer 2015;15(4):e177–87.
36. Wiese D, Stroup AM, Crosbie A, et al. The impact of neighborhood economic and racial inequalities on the spatial variation of breast cancer survival in New Jersey. Cancer Epidemiol Biomarkers Prev 2019;28(12):1958–67.
37. Shariff-Marco S, DeRouen MC, Yang J, et al. Neighborhood archetypes and breast cancer survival in California. Ann Epidemiol 2021;57:22–9.
38. Collin LJ, Gaglioti AH, Beyer KM, et al. Neighborhood-level redlining and lending bias are associated with breast cancer mortality in a large and diverse metropolitan area. Cancer Epidemiol Biomarkers Prev 2021;30(1):53–60.
39. Russell E, Kramer MR, Cooper HL, et al. Residential racial composition, spatial access to care, and breast cancer mortality among women in Georgia. J Urban Health 2011;88(6):1117–29.
40. Jewett PI, Gangnon RE, Elkin E, et al. Geographic access to mammography facilities and frequency of mammography screening. Ann Epidemiol 2018;28(2):65–71.e2.
41. Fan L, Mohile S, Zhang N, et al. Self-reported cancer screening among elderly Medicare beneficiaries: a rural-urban comparison. J Rural Health 2012;28(3):312–9.
42. Khan N, Kaestner R, Salmon JW, et al. Does supply influence mammography screening? Am J Health Behav 2010;34(4):465–75.
43. Lee M, Jenkins WD, Adjei Boakye E. Cancer screening utilization by residence and sexual orientation. Cancer Causes Control 2020;31(10):951–64.
44. Chandak A, Nayar P, Lin G. Rural-urban disparities in access to breast cancer screening: a spatial clustering analysis. J Rural Health 2019;35(2):229–35.
45. Young SG, Ayers M, Malak SF. Mapping mammography in Arkansas: locating areas with poor spatial access to breast cancer screening using optimization models and geographic information systems. J Clin Transl Sci 2020;4(5):437–42.
46. Henry KA, McDonald K, Sherman R, et al. Association between individual and geographic factors and nonadherence to mammography screening guidelines. J Womens Health (Larchmt) 2014;23(8):664–74.
47. Tran L, Tran P. US urban-rural disparities in breast cancer-screening practices at the national, regional, and state level, 2012-2016. Cancer Causes Control 2019;30(10):1045–55.
48. Davis TC, Arnold CL, Rademaker A, et al. Differences in barriers to mammography between rural and urban women. J women's Health (2002) 2012;21(7):748–55.

49. Oeffinger KC, Fontham ET, Etzioni R, et al. Breast cancer screening for women at average risk: 2015 guideline update from the American Cancer Society. Jama 2015;314(15):1599–614.

50. Williams F, Jeanetta S, James AS. Geographical location and stage of breast cancer diagnosis: a systematic review of the literature. J Health Care Poor Underserved 2016;27(3):1357–83.

51. Williams F, Thompson E. Disparity in breast cancer late stage at diagnosis in Missouri: does rural versus urban residence matter? J Racial Ethnic Health Disparities 2016;3(2):233–9.

52. America Cancer Society. . Breast cancer facts & figures 2019-2020. 2019. Available at: https://www.cancer.org/content/dam/cancer-org/research/cancer-facts-and-statistics/breast-cancer-facts-and-figures/breast-cancer-facts-and-figures-2019-2020.pdf.

53. Obeng-Gyasi S, Timsina L, Bhattacharyya O, et al. Breast cancer presentation, surgical management and mortality across the rural-urban continuum in the National Cancer Database. Ann Surg Oncol 2020;27(6):1805–15.

54. Longacre CF, Neprash HT, Shippee ND, et al. Evaluating travel distance to radiation facilities among rural and urban breast cancer patients in the Medicare population. J Rural Health 2020;36(3):334–46.

55. DeCoster RC, Bautista RF Jr, Burns JC, et al. Rural-urban differences in breast reconstruction utilization following oncologic resection. J Rural Health 2020;36(3):347–54.

56. Bauder AR, Gross CP, Killelea BK, et al. The relationship between geographic access to plastic surgeons and breast reconstruction rates among women undergoing mastectomy for cancer. Ann Plast Surg 2017;78(3):324–9.

57. Nash R, Goodman M, Lin CC, et al. State variation in the receipt of a contralateral prophylactic mastectomy among women who received a diagnosis of invasive unilateral early-stage breast cancer in the United States, 2004-2012. JAMA Surg 2017;152(7):648–57.

58. Lizarraga IM, Kahl AR, Jacoby E, et al. Impact of age, rurality and distance in predicting contralateral prophylactic mastectomy for breast cancer in a Midwestern state: a population-based study. Breast Cancer Res Treat 2021. https://doi.org/10.1007/s10549-021-06105-x.

59. Fisher B, Costantino J, Redmond C, et al. Lumpectomy compared with lumpectomy and radiation therapy for the treatment of intraductal breast cancer. N Engl J Med 1993;328(22):1581–6.

60. Andreason M, Zhang C, Onitilo AA, et al. Treatment differences between urban and rural women with hormone receptor-positive early-stage breast cancer based on 21-gene assay recurrence score result. J Community Support Oncol 2015;13(5):195–201.

61. Henley SJAR, Thomas CC, Massetti GM, et al. Invasive cancer incidence, 2004–2013, and deaths, 2006–2015, in nonmetropolitan and metropolitan counties — United States. MMWR Surveill Summ 2017;66(No. SS-1):1–3.

62. Chu QD, Hsieh MC, Chu Y, et al. Do rural patients with operable breast cancer fare worse than urban patients in Louisiana? Results of the Louisiana Cancer Consortium. Surgery 2020;168(4):653–61.

The Impact of Health Delivery Integration on Cancer Outcomes

Vishnukamal Golla, MD, MPH[a,b,c,d,e,]*,
Deborah R. Kaye, MD, MS[b,c,d]

KEYWORDS

- Integrated delivery networks (IDNs) • Value-based care • Cancer care
- Health delivery integration • Alternative payment models (APMs)
- Horizontal integration • Vertical integration • Consolidation

KEY POINTS

- There is significant variation in the degree of integration among integrated delivery networks, which may affect outcomes.
- Integration does not necessarily translate into clinical care coordination.
- Theoretically, health care integration improves costs. However, across many health care settings, integration has shown increased costs with little impact on quality.
- Health care integration's impacts on cancer outcomes and costs are largely mixed.

INTRODUCTION

The American Cancer Society estimates that in 2020 there were ~1.8 million new cancer cases and ~600,000 cancer deaths, making cancer the second leading cause of death in the United States.[1] Cancer-attributed medical care costs are projected to increase by more than 30%, totaling nearly $246 billion by 2030.[2] Health delivery integration, with its emphasis on financial and clinical coordination across the continuum of care, has been proposed as a mechanism to address increasing costs and deficits in quality.[3] In contrast with the fragmentation pervading the US health system, health delivery integration potentially offers patient access to coordinated multidisciplinary teams of health care providers and centers of excellence, and unified electronic medical records and aligned incentives.[4–6]

Examples of health delivery integration include integrated delivery networks (IDNs), vertical integration, horizontal integration, alternative payment models (APMs), and

[a] Duke National Clinician Scholars Program, 200 Morris St, Suite 3400, DUMC Box 104427, Durham, NC 27701, USA; [b] Department of Surgery, Division of Urology, Duke University Medical Center, Durham, NC, USA; [c] Duke Cancer Institute, Durham, NC, USA; [d] Duke-Margolis Policy Center; [e] Durham Veterans Affairs Health Care System, Durham, NC, USA
* Corresponding author. Duke National Clinician Scholars Program, 200 Morris St, Suite 3400, DUMC Box 104427, Durham, NC 27701, USA
E-mail address: vishnukamal.golla@duke.edu

Surg Oncol Clin N Am 31 (2022) 91–108
https://doi.org/10.1016/j.soc.2021.08.003
1055-3207/22/© 2021 Elsevier Inc. All rights reserved.

care delivery models (these are defined later). Although the success of some integrated structures, such as Kaiser and Geisinger Health, have bolstered enthusiasm for health delivery integration, significant heterogeneity exists in the extent of integration for current structures.[7,8] Furthermore, empirical evidence shows that integration has largely been associated with stagnation or declines in quality and higher costs across many disease sites.[9–12] In the context of complex multidisciplinary cancer care, the advantages and potential disadvantages of health delivery integration are emerging with incipient systematic evaluations.

This article begins by detailing the history of health delivery integration. Next, it provides an overview of the practical classifications of integration and their archetypes in our current health care system, including both structural integration and payment models potentially supporting care coordination. In addition, it reports the impact of integration on both quality and cost across the spectrum of cancer care.

Health Delivery Integration

History of integrated delivery networks

Since World War II, the fee-for-service (FFS) model has been the predominant payment model in the US health care system, rewarding volume more than value.[13] This model has created a systemic issue of fragmentation in the US health care system. To combat the deficiencies engendered by fragmentation, large multispecialty group practices began to develop under a single umbrella of common infrastructure and finances.[14] As a result, providers secured better price negotiations with insurers and enhanced patient referrals internally within the group. Practices further consolidated by vertically integrating with several multispecialty groups to promote care coordination. Thus, vertical and horizontal integration laid the groundwork for integrated delivery systems.

Some of these multispecialty groups began accepting fixed payment sums for services. These prepaid group practices gave rise to the concept of health maintenance organizations (HMOs). HMOs served as an alternative for the FFS model and represented early experiments with capitation to restrict health care costs.[15] With capitation, providers were paid a fixed sum per patient, with provider organizations profiting when they delivered services that were less than this fixed sum. In theory, this would spur providers to deliver value-based care. However, gatekeeper tactics, including prior authorizations, and the use of highly restricted networks incited significant backlash, resulting in a decline in HMO enrollment.[16]

However, this emphasis on shifting financial risk and providing incentives laid the groundwork for future health reform. In 2010, President Barack Obama signed into the law the Patient Protection and Affordable Care Act (ACA), driving reform of US health care delivery.[17]

The Centers of Medicare and Medicaid Innovation (CMMI) was established within the ACA as a legislative vehicle to institute innovative payment and service delivery models with the goals of reducing expenditures while enhancing quality.[18] One of the most visible alternative payment approaches by Centers for Medicare and Medicaid Services (CMS) was the 2012 launch of the Accountable Care Organization (ACO) and the Medicare Shared Savings Program (MSSP).[19] In the ACO model, physicians and health care organizations are contracted with the responsibility for both the quality and cost outcomes of a predetermined population of FFS Medicare beneficiaries.[19,20] ACOs are incentivized to deliver cost-effective care by earning shared-savings payments when they reduce per-beneficiary spending benchmarked to historical spending targets. Although ACOs and MSSP were not established specifically for cancer, the diffusions of these models and increased coverage of patients have affected cancer care.[21]

Numerous other APMs and care delivery models have specifically addressed cancer care, including bundled payments, oncology care models, and Patient-centered Medical Homes.

Payers, faced with increasing pressures to contain costs and improve quality, have turned toward such models. This trend has resulted in changed incentives for hospitals and providers as they assume increased financial risk.[22] In addition, there are increasing concerns by independent physicians about competing with larger health systems coupled with an increased desire by younger physicians for a better work/life balance and financial security by joining larger health systems.[10,23] These are some of the many factors driving independent hospitals to join health systems and physicians to transition from being private practice to salaried health system employees.[22] This exodus by independent hospitals and physicians has further spurred the growth of ACOs, APMs, and care delivery models.

ACOs and APMs are frequently formed from integrated hospitals and practice groups, allowing the IDNs to manage their costs of care.[24] Although the concept of IDNs first appeared in the 1930s, they became increasingly prominent in the 1980s and 1990s and more recently showed a strong resurgence.[3,13] There are now more than 980 IDNs across the United States that are heterogeneous in their level of care coordination, integration, and structure.[25] Most of any given region in the United States is dominated by 1 to 3 large health systems, contributing to a highly concentrated hospital market.[26] In cancer care specifically, vertical integration grew sharply after 2010, with ~60% of oncology practices under contract by a hospital or health system compared with 30% in 2010.[27] The different models of health care integration are highlighted next.

Models of Health Delivery Integration

Integrated delivery network
At their core, IDNs are self-contained systems of care that emphasize the cultural values of fiscal accountability and quality across the continuum of care for a patient population. Structurally this integration is substratified into 2 types of integration: horizontal and vertical.

Horizontal integration
Horizontal integration is defined by organizations that acquire or integrate with other organizations providing similar clinical services. For example, when 1 physician group buys another physician's practice.

Vertical integration
In vertical integration, multiple aspects of care are offered by entities that consolidate at different levels of the health care supply chain.[28] This strategy promotes building of IDNs providing the entire gamut of clinical services.[29] Common examples of vertical integration are hospitals that purchase physician groups and those that provide insurance plans. Another highly publicized example is the merger of pharmacy benefit manager CVS and the health insurance company Aetna.

Vertically and/or horizontally integrated systems can participate in APMs and care delivery models designed to improve value. APMs are defined as health care interventions that increase value-based care by altering the financing of care delivery.[30] In cancer care, the most common APMs are ACOs and bundled payments. ACOs are structurally designed so that health care professionals are under the ownership of larger organizations with multiple organizations comprising an ACO. Although these potentially affect cancer care, they predominately focus on primary rather than specialty care.

Bundled payments are defined as APMs that replace traditional FFS with a single payment for an episode of care, and are frequently bundled interventions with private payers.[30] Examples include the Blue Cross Blue Shield (BCBS) of Florida localized prostate cancer bundle; the BCBS of California radiation therapy for breast cancer bundle; and the United Healthcare bundle for management of breast, colon, and lung cancer.[30]

The Oncology Care Model is the most ambitious episode-based alternative payment reform touted by CMMI, with a plan to include 3200 oncology practitioners serving 150,000 beneficiaries.[20] Chemotherapy administration is the trigger event for initiating the bundle payment in the Oncology Care Model.[31] This APM focuses on patients receiving oncological therapy and performance-based payments tied to reductions in Medicare spending.[32]

Care Delivery Model

Care delivery models focus on improving the delivery of care.[30] Commonly used care delivery models in oncology include Patient-centered Medical Homes, where physicians lead care teams in disease management across the disease continuum.

Although these definitions capture the ideal values encompassed in the complex IDN construct, it is critical to understand that there is significant variation in the degree of integration. Furthermore, integration does not necessarily equate to care coordination, and this heterogeneity of integration is partly responsible for the large variations in outcomes across integrated health systems.[33]

Advantages and disadvantages of health delivery integration

Health delivery integration has the theoretic advantage of aligning incentives between all stakeholders (ie, providers, payers, and patients) while delivering a holistic consumer experience. Integration also potentially allows for capitation diversification because of the larger patient and provider pools, reduction in contract costs with payers, lower administrative burdens, and an emphasis on improvement in quality across the continuum of care.[34] In terms of cancer care, vertical integration could potentially mitigate delays in cancer diagnosis and treatment while standardizing the quality of treatment.[35] Furthermore, integration potentially allows for development of infrastructure (eg, electronic medical records) and promotes the attraction of clinical talent.[24]

However, integrated health care also poses significant disadvantages. Evidence shows that both horizontal and vertical integration increase prices and spending, whereas quality remains stagnant or even declines across many disease states.[6,36–39] This finding is in part caused by the increased market share afforded to an integrated health system and success in negotiating higher rates from private insurers,[40,41] leading to shifts to higher-priced hospitals for inpatient admissions, preference for ambulatory facilities, and higher prices to insurers for ancillary services.[29]

Furthermore, APMs are challenging and complex because they define episodes, durations, and beneficiaries in advance. In addition, they have to account for variations in costs across geographic regions, differing disease states, and ever-evolving clinical guidelines.[42] For example, the Oncology Care Model, although touted to improve cancer treatment, has done little to improve the use of value-oriented chemotherapy or radiation regimens.[43] OCM has also fallen short in reducing hospitalizations or emergency department (ED) visits for patients receiving cancer treatment.[44] Furthermore, the care model suffers from an inability to distinguish between different cancer types and rigid bundled costs of care that can limit physicians' use of novel effective therapies.[45,46] These deficiencies leave considerable room for improvement. A new initiative by the CMMI called the Radiation Oncology Model holds some promise by allowing for increased payment predictability and additional flexibility for clinical management of care episodes.[47]

Although there are technical differences between APMs and care delivery models, ideally, they should complement one another. Care delivery models continue to be developed; however, there is considerable difficulty in determining the best payment strategy to support them.

Successes in health delivery integration
As previously mentioned, successes and barriers of cancer care are partially determined by the degree to which health system integration contributes to clinical care coordination.

There are several health delivery integration models that highlight the purported benefits of shifting toward value-based cancer care. Examples of some of the most successful IDNs, APMs, and care delivery models are presented next.

Integrated delivery networks
A. Veterans Health Administration. The Veterans Health Administration (VHA) is one of the largest integrated health systems in the United States, providing care for more than 9 million veterans and ∼3% of cancer cases in the United States.[48,49] The VHA underwent a period of restructuring in the 1990s in which cancer services were realigned. During this process, integrated service networks were developed, including comprehensive cancer centers, local cancer registries, a research partnership with the National Cancer Institute, and a centralized electronic data infrastructure.[50] As a result, the United States Department of Veterans Affairs (VA) has been shown to excel in the screening and diagnosis of cancers with less pronounced racial and ethnic disparity versus non-VA sites of care as well as limiting inappropriate care at the end of life.[51] These successes have been attributed to the integrated system in which veterans receive their care.

B. Kaiser Permanente and Geisinger Health System. Kaiser Permanente and Geisinger Health System are examples of single-entity delivery systems that also include a health plan.[13] These single entities are in an exclusive contractual relationship between providers, insurers, and ancillary partners in all enterprises and are jointly held accountable for care.[52] Both of these examples exemplify the advantages of integration, including the promotion of evidence-based medicine, use of health information technology, and cost controlling by minimizing duplication of services.[8] However, even among these successes, integration has been associated with increases in price and costs.[10,53] Resultant quality of care could also potentially decrease because of reduced competition in the health care market.[54]

Alternative payment models
APMs have shown some successes in improving cancer care, which can vary by specialist engagement. ACOs with more robust urologist engagement are less likely to overtreat men with prostate cancer.[55,56] ACO enrollment has also shown decreased rates of overscreening for breast and prostate cancer and increased rates of appropriate colorectal screening.[57]

Care delivery models
One prominent example of a care delivery is the Community Oncology Medical Home, whose success in reducing emergency room visits and inpatient hospitalizations and maintaining high patient satisfaction may potentially be replicated by the CMS in practices across the country.[58]

Spectrum of Cancer Care

The impacts of health delivery integration on the different phases of cancer care in relation to screening and diagnosis, treatment, end-of-life care, cancer survivorship, and research and clinical trials are discussed next.

Screening and diagnosis

Screening and diagnosis are critical to achieving good cancer outcomes; delays in diagnosis affect survival rates.[59–61] Patient barriers to navigating health care systems, including prolonged wait times and poor referral guidelines, can contribute to delays in diagnosis.[62–64] Integration serves as a systems-level intervention to mitigate these deficiencies by improving access to diagnostic tests and fast-tracking cancer screening.[65–67] Furthermore, a cancer screening program should balance screening with the subsequent risks of overdiagnosis and treatment. To that end, adherence to evidence-based guidelines in cancer screening is critical.

A. Vertical integration. Physician adherence to evidence-based cancer screening and diagnosis for colorectal and cervical cancer improved with vertical integration.[24,68] This improvement was again seen in federally qualified health care systems that monitored the progress of breast, cervical, and colorectal cancer screening, with data showing that colorectal screening increased from 8.6% to 21.2%.[69]

In contrast, some studies show lower rates of colon cancer screening in vertical integration compared with horizontally integrated physician-owned practices.[70] Similarly, after an IDN acquired stand-alone clinics, colorectal and cervical cancer screening rates improved, but breast cancer screening results were mixed.[24,71] However, these studies were not able to elucidate the reasons for these inconsistencies and further research will be needed.

B. Horizontal integration. The impact of horizontal integration largely mirrors that of vertically integrated systems. Horizontally integrated physician practices show higher rates of breast and cervical cancer screening compared with nonintegrated practices.[72]

C. Alternative payment models. The creation of APMs such as bundled payments specifically designed for cancer screening have not been widely adopted. However, there have been several studies exploring the utility and feasibility of bundled payments for cancer screening.[73–77] Real-world application of APMs for this purpose and their impact on cancer screening have not been well elucidated.

ACOs are the primary APM for which the impact on cancer screening has been evaluated. However, the data examined for APMs are largely heterogeneous. In some studies, ACO enrollment was shown to increase screening for prostate or breast cancer.[78] Medicare ACOs showed improvements in the rates of appropriate breast and colorectal screening by targeting only patients who would benefit.[57] However, in other studies, MSSP ACO enrollment had minimal effect on breast, colorectal, or prostate cancer screening rates.[79,80]

D. Care delivery models. More preventive care and consistent clinical visits with a physician increase the likelihood that a patient will undergo cancer screening.[81,82] The largest driver of screening for breast or colon cancer is a preventive health visit.[83] Patient-centered Medical Homes should theoretically excel by emphasizing quality measures that support chronic disease management, use of preventive health services, and, as a result, increased cancer screening rates. However, preliminary data showed little impact on screening for certain malignancies.[84] One limitation for

Patient-centered Medical Homes is when financial incentives focus predominantly on cost savings rather than quality because the benefits of cancer screening are typically seen in the future, with essentially no cost savings in the short term.[85]

Treatment
Integration can affect cancer treatment by mitigating practice variation and maximizing quality of care.

A. **Vertical integration.** Studies show mixed results on the impact of vertical integration on cancer treatment.

Vertical integration's infrastructure potentially allows for the creation of a robust electronic health record, which could optimize cancer treatment. For example, Kaiser Permanente Southern California showed the importance of aromatase inhibitors and tamoxifen in reducing contralateral breast cancer incidence. They then leveraged the electronic health record to improve treatment adherence and to identify women who needed refills.[86,87]

For prostate cancer care, integrated delivery systems showed improved adherence to quality measures.[88] However, in a Medicare claims–based analysis, health care integration was associated with moderate use of prostate cancer treatment but similar rates of overtreatment.[89] This finding suggests that integrated care alone is not enough to mitigate deficiencies in cancer treatment.

In a study that evaluated colon cancer treatment, integrated health systems delivered higher rates of guideline-concordant surgery and chemotherapy, with racial minorities receiving higher rates of evidence-based care and ultimately experiencing better survival.[90]

However, again, data are equivocal, because subsequent studies found that integration did not affect perioperative outcomes in surgical oncology.[91,92] Several explanations exist for the inconsistencies associated with health system integration. As previously mentioned, varying degrees of integration exist among integrated delivery systems. For example, although some systems may have an electronic health record that is fully compatible across systems, many do not; integration may exist primarily in name rather than in a clinical context. Furthermore, system integration does not necessarily translate into care coordination.[91]

B. **Horizontal integration.** The literature specifically addressing the impact of horizontal integration on cancer treatment is sparse. However, 1 study showed that improved provider-to-provider communication resulted in increased guideline-concordant prescription of hematopoietic colony-stimulating factors for management of neutropenia.[93] Thus, theoretically, if horizontal integration improved provider communication, it could result in better cancer outcomes.

C. **Alternative payment models.** Surgeons and oncologists have continued to play a prominent role in developing cancer treatment APMs. Large Urology Group Practice Associations have worked to develop APMs for prostate cancer, and in *Gynecology Oncology*, there have been early efforts to create an APM for endometrial cancer, which is largely treated with surgical resection.[94,95] The implementation of APMs in the Midwest and Georgia, where oncologists received a bonus reimbursement of $350 per month per patient for adherence to treatment guidelines for breast, lung, or colorectal cancer, showed some moderate success.[96]

Although these APMs have theoretic benefits and, in early applications, have been shown to improve cancer treatment outcomes, the data are not yet mature. Therefore, it is difficult to make broad consensus conclusions at this juncture.

Some studies have even shown the opposite, with minimal improvement in cancer treatment outcomes caused by APMs. For example, researchers evaluating the impact of hospitals participating in MSSP on postsurgical cancer outcomes found no difference in perioperative mortality, readmission, or complications compared with control hospitals.[92] Additional studies confirmed that in looking at overall postsurgical outcomes, there was no significant improvement in complications rates, length of stays, and readmission rates in ACO hospitals versus non-ACO hospitals.[92]

These equivocal findings may be in some part caused by a poor level of integration for cancer care specifically within an ACO.[20] Although specialty care such as surgery is a large cost driver for cancer care, specialists are largely not central to the construction of an ACO, with MSSP and ACOs not requiring specialists or surgeons.[97,98]

D. Care delivery models. Examples of care delivery models that have successfully improved cancer outcomes include the Transitional Care Model, the Community Oncology Medical Home, and the Michigan Oncology Medical Home. The Transitional Care Model used an advanced practice nurse well versed in both the patients' and caregivers' care preferences to serve as the primary point of contact following treatment. The primary role of the nurse was to help the patients transition from the hospital to the next site of care (ie, home or a long-term care facility).[99] This model was evaluated in 3 randomized controlled trials and found to reduce all-cause readmission to hospitals and to improve both quality of life and the overall patient care experience.[100]

Both the Community Oncology Medical Home and the Michigan Oncology Medical Home were also effective in reducing ED visits as well as inpatient admissions.[58,101]

These models potentially provide more benefits to patients given that they are patient focused with a high level of integration around clinical care delivery.

End-of-life care

There is strong evidence to support the inclusion of end-of-life care (eg, palliative care) in cancer care with proven benefits in quality of life, symptoms management, and health care system cost savings.[102] Palliative care conversations for patients requiring advanced care have been shown to improve quality of life and reduce health care costs.[103] Other improvements include a reduction in depression, improved survival, and fewer inpatient and intensive care unit (ICU) readmissions.[104] As a result, there has been a notable uptick in the number of palliative programs across the country.[105] However, these programs have only started taking a prominent foothold within integrated health systems.

Vertical integration and horizontal integration. Requiring the collaboration of multiple health professionals, horizontal integration has played a prominent role in improving patients' access to end-of-life cancer care. Patients were previously only eligible for end-of-life care coverage if they were to proceed with hospice, which, unlike palliative care, does not allow them to receive any cancer care treatment. Now, vertically integrated markets such as the VHA have increasingly adopted palliative care.[106] Recently published data showed a higher intensity of care at the end of life in health systems without integration or a cancer focus, a finding that speaks to the potential advantage of integration in improving end-of-life care in patients with cancer.[107]

Alternative payment models and care delivery models. Only within the past 2 years has CMMI begun to include end-of-life care programs in APMs and care delivery models.[108] Accordingly, their impact on cancer care is still not clear. One recent study examining the impact of ACO enrollment showed minimal reduction of aggressive end-of-life care.[109]

The Oncology Care Model is designed to improve end-of-life care by encouraging practices to include a discussion of prognosis for patients with advanced cancer and including hospice enrollment as a quality metric.[103] Early data suggest fewer hospitalizations at end of life as a result of increased use of palliative care specialists.[43]

Another payment model through CMMI is the Medicare Care Choices Model. This APM provides Medicare beneficiaries with qualifying terminal diagnoses to receive covered hospice-level support while forgoing so-called curative therapies.[20] Again, the data on this new payment model are pending.

Cancer survivorship

There are nearly 18 million cancer survivors in the United States, a number that is expected to increase to ~22 million by 2030.[110] Critical to cancer survivorship is continued surveillance, management of late treatment effects, and helping patients navigate financial toxicity following cancer diagnosis.[111] There is a range of cancer survivorship programs primarily based in academic centers.[112] These programs focus on cancer surveillance, prevention of secondary or recurrent malignancies, and treatment of both medical and psychosocial issues.[113] Often these programs also help transition patients from primarily oncologist-driven care to primary care providers, some with special training in oncology and/or cancer survivorship. Given this variability, some proponents argue that integrated health care systems can standardize and improve the value of cancer survivorship programs.

At present, in many survivorship programs, primary care physicians (PCPs) and oncologists use electronic health records to comanage side effects following cancer treatment as well as medical comorbidities. In addition, PCPs can aid in psychological and behavioral counseling, because many cancer survivorship patients continue to have posttreatment anxiety.[114] This interplay between oncologists and PCPs is better achieved in integrated health systems.[115]

However, most cancer survivorship programs at present reside within academic centers, and there are few data on their role within integrated health care.[111,112] This potential but often unrealized integration will be an important component of future policy initiatives when targeting deficiencies within the continuum of cancer care.

Cancer care research and clinical trials

The success of clinical research hinges on linking structure and process measures in order to affect outcomes. For results to be generalizable, they should draw from diverse populations and community-based settings. In this context, integrated delivery systems provide good testing grounds for clinical research interventions.[116] They are theoretically better equipped to disseminate practice changes, including having linked data sources (eg, electronic health records and tumor registries) that facilitate outcomes research. Results originating from integrated systems are potentially more generalizable because of the geographic and population diversity in which the research is done. Evidence derived from integrated health systems has shown accelerated timelines for implementation of standards-of-care clinical guidelines.[117]

In terms of clinical trials, the ACA requires that commercial insurers cover routine costs associated with cancer clinical trial participation. However, the impact the ACA has had on expanding cancer clinical trial access has been impeded by barriers created by health exchanges with constrained options for hospital and provider networks.[118]

The theoretic benefit of research done in these integrated health systems has the potential for exciting applications in the future. For example, research done in the VHA analyzed a flow map for a patient receiving a positive colorectal screening test to time of diagnostic colonoscopy.[49,119] It found structural and process improvements that allowed for more timely receipt of diagnostic colonoscopy, and the results could be generalized from one integrated system to another.

Costs of Cancer Care in Integrated Health Care Systems

The annual cost of cancer care has continued to increase and was expected to reach $173 billion by 2020.[30] An important component of the ACA and its shift toward value-based care was the passing of the Medicare Access and Children's Health Insurance Program Reauthorization Act (MACRA), which supplanted the ACA and allowed further legislation regarding payment and delivery reforms. This value shift was further cemented with the proposed target of linking 50% of FFS payments to value by 2018. Under this legislation, physicians caring for Medicare patients must either participate in APMs or Merit-based Incentive Payment System (MIPS).

In this value shift, cost drivers for cancer have been identified, such as pharmaceutical costs (eg, chemotherapy), poor end-of-life care, increased ED visits, and unnecessary hospitalizations.[120] Anticancer agents and inpatient admissions have largely driven health care spending in this arena.[32] However, end-of-life care has also been a large contributor to costs: nearly one-third of patients with cancer are admitted to an ICU during the last month of life. Meanwhile, hospice care comprises, on average, only 1 week.[120] Furthermore, there has been significant variation in guideline adherence compounded by regional cost variations that could potentially be mitigated with standardization of care through successful integrated health delivery.[121]

Medicare spending and use

Cost analysis of the Physician Group Practice Demonstration, precursor to the MSSP, found annual savings of $721 for patients with cancer. However, most of the cost savings were secondary to reductions in inpatient hospital spending. There were also sizable increases in spending on chemotherapy and cancer-related procedures.[21] The reason for these cost savings are not completely attributable to an integrated health system and could be secondary to differences in risk-adjustment methodology.[122,123]

Episode-based payments can also potentially play a role in curbing cancer costs by reducing variation across regions and practices. By aligning incentives under a single bundled payment, cost reductions could potentially be realized by increasing evidence-based chemotherapy use, improving care coordination, and decreasing hospitalizations and ED visits.[124]

Care delivery models such as patient-centered Medical Homes have been shown to be effective in generating savings as high as 20% in terms of chemotherapy, inpatient, and ED visit costs.[120] Several oncology models that have been trialed also showed cost savings, with some cost reductions as robust as $33 million.[125]

However, the cost savings described in the literature for integrated health care systems are largely inconsistent, varying from cost savings to equal costs to increased spending.[126] In a cross-sectional analysis of a variety of cancer types, receiving a cancer diagnosis within a Medicare ACO did not equate to significantly reduced spending or health care use.[127] This inconsistency, although not clearly delineated, could again be caused by substantial heterogeneity with regard to the extent of integration reported in these articles. This integration at the level of systems may also lack the granularity to respond to the complex needs of patients with cancer.[128]

Market concentration

Health care integration has also brought to light concerns about a form of market concentration that can potentially result in anticompetitive effects on prices as larger health systems consolidate more negotiating leverage with insurers.[54,126] This issue will continue to be evaluated in the coming years as integrated systems' footprint continues to grow within health care markets.

SUMMARY

Although integrated health care has shown some success in improving cancer care, the data remain largely equivocal, limiting the ability to make broad consensus policy statements. Furthermore, robust data show that costs and use may even be worse in integrated systems that dominate local health care markets. A key discussion point is that integration does not necessarily equate to clinical coordination, which might be the true driver behind the success of integrated health care delivery. In addition, challenges exist in aligning clinical care coordination with APMs, which is key for model success. As the various efforts to shift from a fragmented health system to one focused on value continue to be analyzed, care coordination, access to evidence-based cancer care, and overall outcomes for patients will undoubtedly continue to improve.

ACKNOWLEDGMENTS

The authors sincerely acknowledge Dr Robert Berenson for his help in the preparation of this article.

DISCLOSURE

The authors have nothing to disclose.

REFERENCES

1. Siegel RL, Miller KD, Jemal A. Cancer statistics, 2020. CA Cancer J Clin 2020; 70(1):7–30.
2. Mariotto AB, Enewold L, Zhao J, et al. Medical care costs associated with cancer survivorship in the United States. Cancer Epidemiol Biomarkers Prev 2020; 29(7):1304–12.
3. Wenke Hwang P, Jongwha Chang P, Michelle LaClair M, et al. Effects of Integrated Delivery System on Cost and Quality. Am J Manag Care 2013;19(May 2013 5):175–84. Available at: http://www.ajmc.com/journals/issue/2013/2013-1-vol19-n5/effects-of-integrated-delivery-system-on-cost-and-quality.
4. Berwick DM, Nolan TW, Whittington J. The triple aim: Care, health, and cost. Health Aff 2008;27(3):759–69.
5. Fisher ES, Shortell SM. Accountable care organizations: Accountable for what, to whom, and how. JAMA 2010;304(15):1715–6.
6. Burns LR. The U.S healthcare ecosystem: payers, provider, producers. 1st edition. McGraw Hil; 2021.
7. Lee TH, Bothe A, Steele GD. How geisinger structures its physicians' compensation to support improvements in quality, efficiency, and volume. Health Aff 2012;31(9):2068–73.
8. Mchugh MD, Aiken LH, Eckenhoff ME, et al. Achieving kaiser permanente quality. Health Care Manage Rev 2016;41(3):178–88.
9. Gaynor M, Ho K, Town RJ. The industrial organization of health-care markets. J Econ Lit 2015;53(2):235–84.
10. Berenson RA. A physician's perspective on vertical integration. Health Aff 2017; 36(9):1585–90.

11. Morrisey MA, Alexander J, Burns LR, et al. The effects of managed care on physician and clinical integration in hospitals. Med Care 1999;37(4):350–61.

12. O'Mallyey AS, Bond AM, Berenson RA. Rising Hospital Employment of Physicians: Better Quality, Higher Costs?. 2011. Available at: https://www.researchgate.net/publication/51582727. Accessed April 24, 2021.

13. Over V, Alone C, Intervention P, et al. Best Practices and Innovative Healthcare Reform Models. Am J Manag Care 2009;15(10):S300–5.

14. Shiver JM, Cantiello J, Cantiello J. Integrated Healthcare Delivery Models in Era of Reform. In Managing integrated health systems (1st ed., pp. 1–22). Jones & Bartlett Learning 2016. Available at: http://samples.jbpub.com/9781284044492/Chapter1.pdf.

15. Zuvekas SH, Cohen JW. Paying physicians by capitation: Is the past now prologue? Health Aff 2010;29(9):1661–6.

16. Frakt AB, Mayes R. Beyond capitation: How new payment experiments seek to find the "sweet spot" in amount of risk providers and payers bear. Health Aff 2012;31(9):1951–8.

17. Albright HW, Moreno M, Feeley TW, et al. The implications of the 2010 patient protection and affordable care act and the health care and education reconciliation act on cancer care delivery. Cancer 2011;117(8):1564–74.

18. Patient protection and affordable care Act, pub L No. 111–148, 124 Stat 119 §2705. Available at: https://www.congress.gov/111/plaws/publ148/PLAW-111publ148.pdf. Accessed March 14, 2021.

19. Nyweide DJ, Lee W, Cuerdon TT, et al. Association of Pioneer Accountable Care Organizations vs traditional Medicare fee for service with spending, utilization, and patient experience. JAMA 2015;313(21):2152–61.

20. Brooks GA, Hoverman JR, Colla CH. The Affordable Care Act and Cancer Care Delivery. Cancer J 2017;23(3):163–7.

21. Colla CH, Lewis VA, Gottlieb D J, et al. Cancer spending and accountable care organizations: Evidence from the physician group practice demonstration. Healthcare 2013;1(3–4):100–7.

22. Porter ME, Lee TH. The strategy that will fix health care. Harv Bus Rev 2013;91(12):24.

23. Casalino LP, November EA, Berenson RA, et al. Hospital-physician relations: Two tracks and the decline of the voluntary medical staff model. Health Aff 2008;27(5):1305–14.

24. Carlin CS, Dowd B, Feldman R. Changes in Quality of Health Care Delivery after Vertical Integration. Health Serv Res 2015;50(4):1043–68.

25. The Pivotal Role of Healthcare IDNs in Purchasing & Population Health. Available at: https://blog.definitivehc.com/healthcare-idns-population-health. Accessed March 17, 2021.

26. Cooper AZ, Gaynor M. Addressing Hospital Concentration and Rising Consolidation in the United States 1 % Steps. 2018:1-8.

27. Alpert A, Hsi H, Jacobson M. Evaluating The Role Of Payment Policy In Driving Vertical Integration In The Oncology Market. Health Aff 2017;36(4):680–8.

28. Heeringa J, Mutti A, Furukawa MF, et al. Horizontal and vertical integration of health care providers: A framework for understanding various provider organizational structures. Int J Integr Care 2020;20(1):7–22.

29. Robinson JC, Miller K. Total expenditures per patient in hospital-owned and physician-owned physician organizations in California. JAMA 2014;312(16):1663–9.

30. Aviki EM, Schleicher SM, Mullangi S, et al. Alternative payment and care-delivery models in oncology: A systematic review. Cancer 2018;124(16):3293–306.
31. Jackson HA, Walsh B, Abecassis M. A surgeon's guide to bundled payment models for episodes of care. JAMA Surg 2016;151(1):3–4.
32. Rocque GB, Williams CP, Kenzik KM, et al. Where are the opportunities for reducing health care spending within alternative payment models? J Oncol Pract 2018;14(6):e375–83.
33. Mahoney CD, Berard-Collins CM, Coleman R, et al. Effects of an integrated clinical information system on medication safety in a multi-hospital setting. Am J Heal Pharm 2007;64(18):1969–77.
34. Al-Saddique A. Integrated Delivery Systems (IDSs) as a Means of Reducing Costs and Improving Healthcare Delivery. J Heal Commun 2018;3(1):19.
35. Haire K, Burton C, Park R, et al. Integrated Cancer System: a perspective on developing an integrated system for cancer services in London. Lond J Prim Care (Abingdon) 2013;5(1):29–34.
36. Beaulieu ND, Dafny LS, Landon BE, et al. Changes in Quality of Care after Hospital Mergers and Acquisitions. N Engl J Med 2020;382(1):51–9.
37. Cooper Z, Craig SV, Gaynor M, et al. The Price Ain't Right? Hospital Prices and Health Spending on the Privately Insured*. Q J Econ 2019;134(1):51–107.
38. Tsai TC, Jha AK. Hospital consolidation, competition, and quality: Is bigger necessarily better? JAMA 2014;312(1):29–30.
39. Xu T, Wu AW, Makary MA. The potential hazards of hospital consolidation: Implications for quality, access, and price. JAMA 2015;314(13):1337–8.
40. Mitchell JM, Gresenz CR. Documenting Horizontal Integration Among Urologists Who Treat Prostate Cancer. Med Care Res Rev 2020. https://doi.org/10.1177/1077558720980552. 1077558720980552.
41. Capps C, Dranove D, Ody C. Physician Practice Consolidation Driven By Small Acquisitions, So Antitrust Agencies Have Few Tools To Intervene. Health Aff 2017;36(9):1556–63.
42. Kline RM, Muldoon LD, Schumacher HK, et al. Design challenges of an episode-based payment model in oncology: The centers for medicare & medicaid services oncology care model. J Oncol Pract 2017;13(7):e632–44.
43. Associates A, Hassol A, Newes-Adeyi G, et al. Evaluation of the Oncology Care Model: Performance Periods 1-3 Contract #HHSM-500-2014-000261 T0003 PREPARED FOR: AUTHORS: ACKNOWLEDGMENTS.; 2020. Available at: https://innovation.cms.gov/data-and-reports/2020/ocm-evaluation-annual-report-2-appendices.
44. Bower JT, Scott CA, Mooney KH, et al. The CMS Oncology Care Model Is Falling Short Of Its Promise. Could Oncology Hospital At Home Be The Remedy? | Health Affairs. Health Affairs. 2020. Available at: https://www.healthaffairs.org/do/10.1377/hblog20201221.830917/full/. Accessed April 14, 2021.
45. Diaz M. THE ONCOLOGY CARE MODEL 2.0.; 2019. Available at: https://communityoncology.org/wp-content/uploads/2019/06/COA-PTAC.pdf.
46. Thomas CA, Ward JC. The Oncology Care Model: A Critique. Am Soc Clin Oncol Educ B 2016;36:e109–14.
47. Radiation Oncology Model | CMS Innovation Center. Available at: https://innovation.cms.gov/innovation-models/radiation-oncology-model. Accessed April 25, 2021.
48. Jiang CY, El-Kouri NT, Elliot D, et al. Telehealth for Cancer Care in Veterans: Opportunities and Challenges Revealed by COVID. JCO Oncol Pract 2021;17(1):22–9.

49. Jackson GL, Powell AA, Ordin DL, et al. Developing and sustaining quality improvement partnerships in the VA: The colorectal cancer care collaborative. J Gen Intern Med 2010;25(SUPPL. 1):38–43.

50. Wilson NJ, Kizer KW. Oncology management by the "new" veterans health administration. Cancer 1998;82(10 SUPPL):2003–9.

51. O'Hanlon C, Huang C, Sloss E, et al. Comparing VA and Non-VA Quality of Care: A Systematic Review. J Gen Intern Med 2017;32(1):105–21.

52. Are You a Covered Entity? | CMS. Available at: https://www.cms.gov/Regulations-and-Guidance/Administrative-Simplification/HIPAA-ACA/AreYouaCoveredEntity. Accessed April 24, 2021.

53. Berenson R. Addressing pricing power in integrated delivery: The limits of antitrust. J Health Polit Policy L 2015;40(4):711–44.

54. Burns LR, Goldsmith JC, Sen A. Horizontal and vertical integration of physicians: A tale of two tails. Adv Health Care Manag 2013;15:39–117.

55. Modi PK, Kaufman SR, Borza T, et al. Variation in prostate cancer treatment and spending among Medicare shared savings program accountable care organizations. Cancer 2018;124(16):3364–71.

56. Borza T, Kaufman SR, Yan P, et al. Early effect of Medicare Shared Savings Program accountable care organization participation on prostate cancer care. Cancer 2018;124(3):563–70.

57. Resnick MJ, Graves AJ, Thapa S, et al. Medicare accountable care organization enrollment and appropriateness of cancer screening. JAMA Intern Med 2018;178(5):648–54.

58. Waters TM, Webster JA, Stevens LA, et al. Community oncology medical homes: Physician-driven change to improve patient care and reduce costs. J Oncol Pract 2015;11:462–7.

59. Foot C, Harrison T. How to Improve Cancer Survival: Explaining England's Relatively Poor Rates - The King's Fund, June 2011.; 2011.

60. Henley SJ, King JB, German RR, et al. Surveillance of Screening-Detected Cancers (Colon and Rectum, Breast, and Cervix) — United States, 2004–2006. Morbidity and Mortality Weekly Report. 2010. Available at: https://www.cdc.gov/mmwr/preview/mmwrhtml/ss5909a1.htm. Accessed March 25, 2021.

61. Tørring ML, Frydenberg M, Hansen RP, et al. Time to diagnosis and mortality in colorectal cancer: A cohort study in primary care. Br J Cancer 2011;104(6):934–40.

62. Andersen RS, Vedsted P, Olesen F, et al. Does the organizational structure of health care systems influence care-seeking decisions? A qualitative analysis of Danish cancer patients' reflections on care-seeking. Scand J Prim Health Care 2011;29:144–9.

63. Simon AE, Waller J, Robb K, et al. Patient delay in presentation of possible cancer symptoms: The contribution of knowledge and attitudes in a population sample from the United Kingdom. Cancer Epidemiol Biomarkers Prev 2010;19(9):2272–7.

64. Davies E, van der Molen B, Cranston A. Using clinical audit, qualitative data from patients and feedback from general practitioners to decrease delay in the referral of suspected colorectal cancer. J Eval Clin Pract 2007;13(2):310–7.

65. Olesen F, Hansen RP, Vedsted P. Delay in diagnosis: The experience in Denmark. Br J Cancer 2009;101(2):S5–8.

66. Molassiotis A. The UK and Denmark are still the countries with low all-cancer survival in Europe. Eur J Oncol Nurs 2007;11(5):383–4.

67. Neal RD. Do diagnostic delays in cancer matter? Br J Cancer 2009;101(2): S9–12.
68. Weeks WB, Gottlieb DJ, Nyweide DJ, et al. Higher Health Care Quality And Bigger Savings Found At Large Multispecialty Medical Groups. Health Aff 2010;29(5):991–7.
69. Davis T, Arnold C, Rademaker A, et al. Improving colon cancer screening in community clinics. Cancer 2013;119(21):3879–86.
70. Kralewski J, Dowd B, Knutson D, et al. The relationships of physician practice characteristics to quality of care and costs. Health Serv Res 2015;50(3):710–29.
71. Cole AP, Krasnova A, Ramaswamy A, et al. Prostate cancer in the medicare shared savings program: are Accountable Care Organizations associated with reduced expenditures for men with prostate cancer? Prostate Cancer Prostatic Dis 2019;22(4):593–9.
72. Mehrotra A, Epstein AM, Rosenthal MB. Do integrated medical groups provide higher-quality medical care than individual practice associations? Ann Intern Med 2006;145(11):826–33.
73. Hughes DR, Jiang M, Mcginty G, et al. An Empirical Framework for Breast Screening Bundled Payments. J Am Coll Radiol 2017;14:17–23.
74. Fleming MM, Hughes DR, Golding LP, et al. Digital Breast Tomosynthesis Implementation: Considerations for Emerging Breast Cancer Screening Bundled Payment Models. J Am Coll Radiol 2019;16(7):902–7.
75. Ketover SR, Charles Accurso A. Proposal for a physician-focused payment model: comprehensive colonoscopy advanced alternative payment model for colorectal cancer screening. Diagnosis and Surveillance; 2016.
76. Brill JV, Jain R, Margolis PS, et al. A bundled payment framework for colonoscopy performed for colorectal cancer screening or surveillance. Gastroenterology 2014;146(3):849–53.e9.
77. Silva E. Lung cancer screening as a predictor of future alternative payment models. J Am Coll Radiol 2014;11(11):1022.
78. Meyer CP, Krasnova A, Sammon JD, et al. Accountable care organizations and the use of cancer screening. Prev Med (Baltim) 2017;101:15–7.
79. Resnick MJ, Graves AJ, Gambrel RJ, et al. The association between Medicare accountable care organization enrollment and breast, colorectal, and prostate cancer screening. Cancer 2018;124(22):4366–73.
80. Luckenbaugh AN, Hollenbeck BK, Kaufman SR, et al. Impact of Accountable Care Organizations on Diagnostic Testing for Prostate Cancer. Urology 2018; 116:68–75.
81. Fenton JJ, Cai Y, Weiss NS, et al. Delivery of cancer screening: How important is the preventive health examination? Arch Intern Med 2007;167(6):580–5.
82. Bindman AB, Grumbach K, Osmond D, et al. Primary care and receipt of preventive services. J Gen Intern Med 1996;11(5):269–76.
83. Ruffin IVMT, Gorenflo DW, Woodman B. Predictors of Screening for Breast, Cervical, Colorectal, and Prostatic Cancer among Community-Based Primary Care Practices. J Am Board Fam Pract 2000;13(1):1–10.
84. Hong YR, Xie Z, Mainous AG, et al. Patient-Centered Medical Home and Up-To-Date on Screening for Breast and Colorectal Cancer. Am J Prev Med 2020; 58(1):107–16.
85. Sarfaty M, Wender R, Smith R. Promoting cancer screening within the patient centered medical home. CA Cancer J Clin 2011;61(6):397–408.
86. Chlebowski RT, Kim J, Haque R. Adherence to endocrine therapy in breast cancer adjuvant and prevention settings. Cancer Prev Res 2014;7(4):378–87.

87. Haque R, Ahmed SA, Fisher A, et al. Effectiveness of aromatase inhibitors and tamoxifen in reducing subsequent breast cancer. Cancer Med 2012;1(3): 318–27.

88. Herrel LA, Kaufman SR, Yan P, et al. Healthcare Integration and quality among men with prostate cancer. J Urol 2018;197(1):55–60.

89. Hollenbeck BK, Bierlein MJ, Kaufman SR, et al. Implications of evolving delivery system reforms for prostate cancer care. Am J Manag Care 2016;22(9):569–75.

90. Rhoads KF, Patel MI, Ma Y, et al. How do integrated health care systems address racial and ethnic disparities in colon cancer? J Clin Oncol 2015; 33(8):854–60.

91. Li J, Ye Z, Dupree JM, et al. Association of delivery system integration and outcomes for major cancer surgery. Physiol Behav 2016;176(1):100–6.

92. Herrel LA, Norton EC, Hawken SR, et al. Early impact of Medicare accountable care organizations on cancer surgery outcomes. Cancer 2016;122(17): 2739–46.

93. Bennett CL, Weeks JA, Somerfield MR, et al. Use of hematopoietic colony-stimulating factors: Comparison of the 1994 and 1997 American Society of Clinical Oncology Surveys regarding ASCO clinical practice guidelines. J Clin Oncol 1999;17(11):3676–81.

94. Kapoor DA, Shore ND, Kirsh GM, et al. The LUGPA Alternative Payment Model for Initial Therapy of Newly Diagnosed Patients With Organ-confined Prostate Cancer: Rationale and Development. Rev Urol 2017;19(4):235–45.

95. Liang MI, Aviki EM, Wright JD, et al. Society of gynecologic oncology future of physician payment reform task force: Lessons learned in developing and implementing surgical alternative payment models. Gynecol Oncol 2020;156(3): 701–9.

96. Wen L, Divers C, Lingohr-Smith M, et al. Improving Quality of Care in Oncology Through Healthcare Payment Reform. Vol 24. Available at: www.ajmc.com. Accessed March 21, 2021.

97. Hawken SR, Ryan AM, Miller DC. Surgery and medicare shared savings program accountable care organizations. JAMA Surg 2016;151(1):5–6.

98. Dupree JM, Patel K, Singer SJ, et al. Attention to surgeons and surgical care is largely missing from early medicare accountable care organizations. Health Aff 2014;33(6):972–9.

99. Van Cleave JH, Smith-Howell E, Naylor MD. Achieving a High-Quality Cancer Care Delivery System for Older Adults: Innovative Models of Care. Semin Oncol Nurs 2016;32(2):122–33.

100. Naylor MD. Advancing high value transitional care: The central role of nursing and its leadership. Nurs Adm Q 2012;36(2):115–26.

101. Colligan EM, Ewald E, Ruiz S, et al. Innovative oncology care models improve end-of-life quality, reduce utilization and spending. Health Aff 2017;36(3): 433–40.

102. Wiencek C, Coyne P. Palliative Care Delivery Models. Semin Oncol Nurs 2014; 30(4):227–33.

103. Zhang B, Wright AA, Huskamp HA, et al. Health care costs in the last week of life associations with End-of-life conversations. Arch Intern Med 2009;169(5):480–8.

104. Smith G, Bernacki R, Block SD. The role of palliative care in population management and accountable care organizations. J Palliat Med 2015;18(6):486–94.

105. Morrison RS, Maroney-Galin C, Kralovec PD, et al. The growth of palliative care programs in United States hospitals. J Palliat Med 2005;8(6):1127–34.

106. Hughes MT, Smith TJ. The Growth of Palliative Care in the United States. Annu Rev Public Heal 2014;35:459–75.

107. Herrel LA, Zhu Z, Griggs JJ, et al. Association Between Delivery System Structure and Intensity of End-of-Life Cancer Care. JCO Oncol Pract 2020;16(7): e590–600.

108. New Medicare Alternative Payment Models: Options and Opportunities for Hospices and Palliative Care Programs | National Coalition For Hospice and Palliative Care. Available at: https://www.nationalcoalitionhpc.org/event/new-medicare-alternative-payment-models-options-and-opportunities-for-hospices-and-palliative-care-programs/. Accessed April 3, 2021.

109. Kim H, Keating NL, Perloff JN, et al. Aggressive Care near the End of Life for Cancer Patients in Medicare Accountable Care Organizations. J Am Geriatr Soc 2019;67(5):961–8.

110. Statistics, Graphs and Definitions | Division of Cancer Control and Population Sciences (DCCPS). Available at: https://cancercontrol.cancer.gov/ocs/statistics. Accessed March 30, 2021.

111. Chubak J, Tuzzio L, Hsu C, et al. Providing care for cancer survivors in integrated health care delivery systems: practices, challenges, and research opportunities. J Oncol Pract 2012;8(3):184–9.

112. Oeffinger KC, McCabe MS. Models for delivering survivorship care. J Clin Oncol 2006;24(32):5117–24.

113. Oeffinger KC, Argenbright KE, Levitt GA, et al. Models of Cancer Survivorship Health Care: Moving Forward. Am Soc Clin Oncol Educ B 2014;34:205–13.

114. Sada YH, Street RL, Singh H, et al. Primary care and communication in shared cancer care: A qualitative study. Am J Manag Care 2011;17(4):259–65. Available at:/pmc/articles/PMC3693186/. Accessed March 21, 2021.

115. Jacobsen PB. Clinical practice guidelines for the psychosocial care of cancer survivors. Cancer 2009;115(S18):4419–29.

116. Mooney KH, Beck SL, Friedman RH, et al. Automated monitoring of symptoms during ambulatory chemotherapy and oncology providers' use of the information: A randomized controlled clinical trial. Support Care Cancer 2014;22(9): 2343–50.

117. Ramirez A, Perez-Stable E, Penedo F, et al. Reducing time-to-treatment in underserved Latinas with breast cancer: The Six Cities Study. Cancer 2014; 120(5):752–60.

118. Kehl KL, Liao KP, Krause TM, et al. Access to accredited cancer hospitals within federal exchange plans under the affordable care act. J Clin Oncol 2017;35(6): 645–51.

119. Powell AA, Gravely AA, Ordin DL, et al. Timely Follow-Up of Positive Fecal Occult Blood Tests Strategies Associated with Improvement. Am J Prev Med 2009. https://doi.org/10.1016/j.amepre.2009.05.013.

120. Knight D. Integrate Care Models are the Future of Oncology. 2017.

121. Ellimoottil C, Li J, Ye Z, et al. Episode-based Payment Variation for Urologic Cancer Surgery. Urology 2018;111:78–85.

122. Ibrahim AM, Dimick JB, Sinha SS, et al. Association of coded severity with readmission reduction after the hospital readmissions reduction program. JAMA Intern Med 2018;178(2):83–5.

123. Pope GC, Michael Trisolini M, John Kautter M, et al. Physician Group Practice (PGP) Demonstration Design Report.; 2002.

124. Kline RM, Bazell C, Smith E, et al. Centers for Medicare and Medicaid Services: Using an episode-based payment model to improve oncology care. J Oncol Pract 2015;11(2):114–6.
125. Newcomer LN, Gould B, Page RD, et al. Changing physician incentives for affordable, quality cancer care: Results of an episode payment model. J Oncol Pract 2014;10(5):322–6.
126. Machta RM, Maurer KA, Jones DJ, et al. A systematic review of vertical integration and quality of care, efficiency, and patient-centered outcomes. Health Care Manage Rev 2019;44(2):159–73.
127. Lam MB, Figueroa JF, Zheng J, et al. Spending among patients with cancer in the first 2 years of accountable care organization participation. J Clin Oncol 2018;36(29):2955–60.
128. Kaye DR, Min HS, Norton EC, et al. System-level health-care integration and the costs of cancer care across the disease continuum. J Oncol Pract 2018;14(3): e149–57.

Disparities in Genetic Testing for Heritable Solid-Tumor Malignancies

Jacquelyn Dillon, MS[a], Foluso O. Ademuyiwa, MD, MPH, MSCI[b],
Megan Barrett, MD[c], Haley A. Moss, MD[c,d],
Elizabeth Wignall, MS[e], Carolyn Menendez, MD[a,e],
Kevin S. Hughes, MD[f], Jennifer K. Plichta, MD, MS[a,g],*

KEYWORDS

- Genetic testing • Germline genetic testing • Disparities • Hereditary cancer

KEY POINTS

- Genetic testing offers providers a potentially life saving tool for identifying and intervening in high-risk individuals.
- Disparities in receipt of genetic testing have been consistently demonstrated and undoubtedly have significant implications for populations not receiving the standard of care.
- If correctly used, genetic testing may play a role in decreasing health disparities among individuals of different races and ethnicities.
- However, if genetic testing continues to revolutionize cancer care while being disproportionately distributed, it also has the potential to widen the existing mortality gap between various racial and ethnic populations.

INTRODUCTION

Advances in cancer genetics, targeted therapies, and risk reduction strategies have greatly transformed the field of oncology. Genetic testing is now an essential tool in the identification of high-risk individuals. In particular, testing for germline genetic variants that predispose carriers to solid tumor malignances including breast, ovarian, uterine, prostate, and colorectal cancers have become increasingly available over

[a] Department of Surgery, Duke University Medical Center, Durham, NC, USA; [b] Department of Medicine, Washington University School of Medicine, St Louis, MO, USA; [c] Department of Obstetrics & Gynecology, Duke University Medical Center, Durham, NC, USA; [d] Duke Cancer Institute, Durham, NC, USA; [e] Clinical Cancer Genetics, Duke Cancer Institute, Durham, NC, USA; [f] Surgical Oncology, Massachusetts General Hospital, Boston, MA, USA; [g] Department of Population Health Sciences, Duke University Medical Center, Durham, NC, USA
* Corresponding author. DUMC 3513, Durham, NC 27710.
E-mail address: jennifer.plichta@duke.edu
Twitter: @haleyarden1 (H.A.M.); @CSMenendez (C.M.); @JenniferPlichta (J.K.P.)

Surg Oncol Clin N Am 31 (2022) 109–126
https://doi.org/10.1016/j.soc.2021.08.004
1055-3207/22/© 2021 Elsevier Inc. All rights reserved.

the last 25 years.[1] Sequencing and deletion/duplication analysis of cancer predisposition genes can guide future screening practices, disease-modifying surgery, risk-reducing medication administration, and treatment options for those already diagnosed with cancer. However, disparities in receipt of genetic testing have been consistently demonstrated across numerous studies and undoubtedly have significant implications for those populations not receiving the standard of care.

CURRENT GUIDELINES ON GENETIC TESTING

Apart from newborn screening tests, which are nearly universal in the United States and do not include any screening for cancer predisposition,[2] there are no agencies that recommend universal germline genetic screening for individuals without risk factors. The concept of universal cancer genetic testing has been considered, and testing among all patients with solid tumors, compared with targeted testing based on clinical guidelines, suggests a possible survival benefit,[3] particularly as some risk-reducing surgeries and/or management strategies may improve survival outcomes.[4–7] However, current guidelines attempt to weigh the potential benefits of universal screening against the risks of testing including the potential for overdiagnosis, psychological distress, and financial burden, with the result being that testing is only recommended when the risk of mutation is high. Current guidelines on who should receive genetic testing are typically cancer dependent and vary across organizations. The most commonly referenced guidelines are those from the United States Preventative Services Task Force,[8] the National Comprehensive Cancer Network (NCCN),[9] and the American Society of Clinical Oncology[10] for genetic testing for various cancer types. However, other organizations including the American Society of Breast Surgeons (ASBrS),[11] the American College of Obstetrics and Gynecology,[12] the Society of Gynecologic Oncology,[13] the American Urologic Association,[14] the American College of Gastroenterology,[15] the American College of Medical Genetics,[16] and others have additional cancer-specific screening guidelines. The variety of recommendations among academic agencies leaves room for physician interpretation and potential bias in referral patterns and recommendations, which can amplify preexisting disparities.

PHYSICIAN AND HEALTH CARE PROVIDER ROLES

Current NCCN guidelines recommend that genetic counseling and testing be performed by a "genetic counselor, medical geneticist, oncologist, surgeon, oncology nurse, or other health professional with expertise and experience in cancer genetics."[9] However, patients must first be identified and, if point-of-care testing is not available, referred for testing. A recent study by Chapman-Davis and colleagues found that genetic testing is recommended most commonly by subspecialty oncologists and surgical oncologists, often at the time of a cancer diagnosis. More recently, a greater percentage of referrals are made by internal medicine, family medicine, and obstetrics and gynecology physicians.[17] Among oncologists, at least 79% have discussed genetic testing with their patients, and 76% have recommended consultation with a genetic counselor.[18] However, identifying patients with a pathogenic germline mutation in a cancer predisposing gene *after* a cancer diagnosis may be considered a failure in prevention.[19] Aside from oncologists, studies have shown that up to 60% of primary care providers (PCPs) have ordered genetic tests related to both cancer and non-cancer diseases and 74% have referred their patients for testing, although these numbers were significantly lower for minority-serving physicians (54% and 63%, respectively, for PCPs with >50% minority patients).[20] Furthermore, a 2010 survey of patients undergoing genetic testing indicated that patients expect their PCP to play a role in risk identification and genetic referral; patients also desire PCP support in interpreting genetic screening results.[21] As genetic testing continues to expand, it will be critical for most of the providers who provide direct patient care to be able to identify appropriate patients for genetic counseling and possibly genetic testing.

POPULATION-BASED GENETIC VARIANTS

The distribution of genetic variants across different populations is not equal, and therefore, certain populations may be at higher risk than others for developing genetically predisposed solid tumors. One well-known group at higher risk for multiple genetic syndromes are people of Ashkenazi Jewish descent. Individuals with this heritage are recommended to undergo heightened screening for certain genetic diseases.[22] More recently, lesser known, high-risk populations have also been discovered. A 2017 study by Caswell-Jin and colleagues examined multiple gene sequencing in a diverse group of 1483 volunteers and found that genetic mutations differed slightly by race and ethnicity. Specifically, a pathogenic CHEK2 mutation was more prominent in Whites compared with non-Whites (3.8% vs 1.0%; $P = .002$).[23] In BRCA1/2 sequencing, a 2015 study by Pal and colleagues identified an almost 2-fold higher BRCA1/2 mutation prevalence in young Black women compared with young White women.[24] Similarly, in a study of patients with breast cancer diagnosed at the age of 50 years or younger between 2007 and 2017, non-Hispanic Blacks and Whites had the highest frequency of pathogenic and likely pathogenic variants (18.2% and 16.3%, respectively, compared with 8.2% in Asians and 7.9% in Hispanics), whereas Asians and Hispanics had the highest frequency of variants of uncertain significance (VUSs, 21.9% and 19%, respectively, compared with 13.6% in non-Hispanic Blacks and 8.7% in non-Hispanic Whites).[25] Another study of 77,900 women with breast cancer and matched controls examined 12 genetic variants (*ATM, BARD1, BRCA1, BRCA2, BRIP1, CDH1, CHEK2, PALB2, PTEN, RAD51C, RAD51D, TP53*) related to breast cancer, and this group similarly noted an unequal distribution of variants among different populations.[26] Interestingly, they also found that pathogenic variants in certain populations did not confer a higher risk of cancer. For example, Blacks and Asians with specific CHEK2 mutations did not have an increased breast cancer risk, nor did Asian carriers of certain pathogenic ATM variants,[26] although this likely requires further study to verify these findings. These data again highlight the critical importance of diversity in research populations.

In general, higher rates of VUSs have been consistently documented in non-White patients, which is often attributed to the underrepresentation of minority populations in genetic research.[27,28] This lack of diversity is common in many large-scale studies on genetic testing, where White groups comprise most of the study populations (**Table 1**). Unfortunately, some providers lack the education necessary to manage patients with VUSs,[29] and this may contribute to some of the observed disparities among populations with higher rates of VUSs.[30] However, many educational opportunities exist to improve one's knowledge related to genetic testing,[31] and such resources will certainly continue to expand.

TRENDS IN DISPARITY

It is well documented that individuals in underserved populations have poorer health outcomes. Race and ethnicity remain independent predictive factors in many health care settings, even when all other demographic factors have been adjusted.[32] Additional factors including socioeconomic status, geographic location, age, insurance

Table 1
Representation of various races and ethnicities in select larger studies (published in 2015–2021) on germline genetic testing related to cancer risk

Publication Year & First Author	Primary Country of Population and/ or Company	Study Population (N)	% White, Caucasian, European (%)	% Black, African American, African (%)	% Hispanic, Latin American (%)	% Asian (%)	% Mixed, Other, Unknown (%)
Hu et al,[50] 2021	USA (CARRIERS Consortium)	64,791	75.0	14	4.9	4.4	1.7
LaDuca et al,[93] 2019	USA (Ambry)	165,024	64.0	6.5	6.0	4.2	19.3
Kurian et al,[59] 2019	USA (SEER)	83,086	62.3	11.5	14.1	11.8	0.3
Couch et al,[94] 2017	USA (Ambry)	65,057	65.0	6.2	5.8	4.0	19.0
Buys et al,[95] 2017	USA (Myriad)	35,409	51.5	7.1	7.1	3.4	30.9
Tung et al,[96] 2015	USA (Myriad)	2158	58.1	5.2	3.9	2.3	30.5
Desmond et al,[97] 2015	USA (3 academic medical centers)	1046	85.4	1.6	3.5	4.7	4.8

coverage, health literacy, and level of medical mistrust can also drive disparities. In cancer care, these factors influence patient outcomes in most solid tumor malignancies. For example, Black and White women have similar rates of breast cancer diagnoses, with Black women having slightly lower incidence; however, Black women are more likely to die of breast cancer compared with their White counterparts.[33] Similarly, Black men are twice as likely to die of prostate cancer compared with Whites, and highly educated individuals are less likely to die prematurely of colorectal cancer compared with less educated counterparts.[33]

The associations between cancer care and disparities in outcomes are numerous and complex. Barriers include limited access to medical care, limited access to transportation, lack of insurance coverage, and language barriers.[34] Beyond these, delays exist in the dissemination of advances in medical knowledge and care to underserved populations.[34] Furthermore, additional factors including health literacy and medical mistrust may influence which patients will undergo recommended treatment or testing. A survey study by Morris and colleagues demonstrated that individuals with low health literacy were more likely to avoid doctor appointments, more likely to report limited knowledge about tests, and less likely to seek medical information from a resource other than their physician.[35] Once identified and defined, removing these barriers will require significant effort at the level of the provider, the health care system, and the community, in order to truly affect change.

DISPARITIES IN GENETIC TESTING

With regard to germline genetic testing, additional unique obstacles related to family history, perceived cost, and access to testing likely introduce genetics referral bias, whereas patient mistrust in the potential mishandling of genetic information has been identified as a major factor in testing adherence.[36] Because family history of cancer is often considered an important factor in genetic testing eligibility, individuals who do not know their biological family's medical history are less likely to qualify for testing. In a study of greater than 43,000 women presenting for screening mammography, the number of paternal family histories was significantly lower than that of maternal family histories of cancer,[37] which may be related to patient reporting and/or data collection, but regardless, would affect a woman's estimated cancer risk. Furthermore, a study seeking to identify patients with hereditary nonpolyposis colon cancers (HNPCC) and familial adenomatous polyposis (FAP) found that unknown paternal history was higher among Black individuals.[38] These gaps in family history may decrease the accuracy of risk assessment models and widen the disparities. In addition, minority and lower socioeconomic status (SES) populations are also less likely to have access to appropriate medical care, and familial cancers are historically underdiagnosed in these groups.[34]

Perceived cost can also be a barrier for individuals considering genetic testing, particularly those with low SES. However, the direct cost of genetic testing has dramatically decreased in recent years, with current costs ranging from $250 to more than $1000.[39] Third-party insurance and Medicare often cover testing for familial cancer syndromes, particularly in those with a cancer diagnosis.[40] Although few patients decline genetic testing due to cost, retrospective analyses have shown that perceived cost may influence a physician's decision to refer for genetic testing.[40–42] Regardless, because not all medical facilities have the infrastructure for genetic testing, patients may experience difficulties with transportation, access, and indirect costs, particularly for those in rural settings.[43] However, with the recent increase in telehealth utilization and shift toward telegenetics (where counseling is done by video or phone and kits are mailed to patients homes), some of these barriers may be drastically reduced, and the outcomes are expected to be equivalent to in-person genetics-related care.[44]

Health literacy and medical mistrust are also significant factors driving diversity in genetic testing. Minority and low-SES populations may have less access to educational materials and may be less knowledgeable about genetic testing.[35,45,46] Furthermore, because of historical instances of mistreatment in the medical system, racial and ethnic minorities have increased rates of medical mistrust and higher levels of concern regarding the misuse of genetic information, which are some of the most common reasons cited for declining genetic testing.[46,47]

Breast Cancer

Breast cancer is the most common noncutaneous cancer in women, and the second leading cause of cancer-related mortality in the United States.[48] Although most of the breast cancers are associated with de novo somatic mutations, approximately 5% to 10% of breast cancers are attributed to a hereditary germline variant.[34] Currently, at least 12 guideline-designated breast cancer-related genes have been identified, including *ATM, BARD1, BRCA1, BRCA2, CDH1, CHEK2, NBN, NF1, PALB2, PTEN, STK11,* and *TP53.*[9,49,50] Patients with an identified variant may be offered increased breast cancer screening,[9,51] and some may also consider risk-reducing mastectomy, which has been shown to decrease the risk of breast cancer in affected individuals by 90% to 95%.[52,53] Carriers of *BRCA1/2* pathogenic variants are also eligible for poly (ADP-ribose) polymerase (PARP) inhibitor chemotherapy for advanced HER2-negative disease.[49] The availability of increased surveillance, risk-reducing surgery, and targeted chemotherapy can greatly decrease morbidity and mortality.[54–56] To effectively use these tools, identification of at-risk individuals is paramount.

Unfortunately, disparities persist in referral patterns and completion of genetic testing. A retrospective study of 723 patients in a single hospital system (2015–2018) showed that physician referral rates varied significantly by race.[57] In women who met NCCN criteria for breast cancer–related genetic counseling, 75.7% of non-Hispanic Black women were referred compared with 92.7% of non-Hispanic White patients (<0.001). Of patients referred, there was no difference in the uptake of counseling by race. Notably, however, referral patterns did differ significantly by employment status (employed 90.1% vs unemployed 72.3% vs unknown 57.1%; P value<.01) but did not significantly differ based on Medicaid status in this study (P value = 09).[57] A similar study of 1622 women aged 50 years or younger and diagnosed with breast cancer between 2009 and 2012 found that physician-provider discussions about genetic testing were 16 times less likely to occur with Black woman compared with White women (P<.0001) and nearly twice less likely to occur with Spanish-speaking Hispanic women (P = .04) compared with English-speaking, non-Hispanic women.[58] A larger study of 77,085 patients diagnosed with breast cancer between 2013 and 2014 and in which 24.1% underwent genetic testing found that testing decreased with increasing age, and individuals living in poorer communities were less likely to receive testing.[59] However, this study did not find differences in testing rates among different races or ethnicities.[59]

In addition to disparities in referral rates, differences are also observed in the indications for referral. In a study of 1666 patients, non-Hispanic Whites were more likely to be referred due to a family history of cancer compared with all other ethnicities, and non-Hispanic Blacks, Hispanics, and Asians were more likely to be referred due to a personal history of cancer (P<.001).[17] For women diagnosed with a high-risk germline variant before a cancer diagnosis, some may consider risk-reducing mastectomies, in accordance with national guidelines.[9] Interestingly, in a cohort of 90 *BRCA* pathogenic variant carriers, Hispanic and non-Hispanic White women were more likely to undergo risk-reducing surgery compared with Black women.[17] Taken together, these data suggest not only that minority women are less likely to be referred for genetic testing based on family history but also that high-risk minority women are less likely to undergo risk-reducing surgery, although some of these differences may be related to cultural preferences, as risk-reducing mastectomy rates have also been shown to vary across countries from around the world.[60]

Gynecologic Cancer

Ovarian cancer represents 4% of all women's cancers worldwide and is the leading cause of gynecologic cancer death.[34] Approximately 25% of high-grade, nonmucinous epithelial ovarian cancers have an underlying hereditary cause,[61] and pathogenic germline variants that increase one's risk of ovarian cancer include *BRCA1, BRCA2, BRIP1, PALB2, TP53, PTEN, RAD51 C, RAD51D*, and *STK11*.[9,61] Although referral rates for genetic testing are increasing for women with ovarian cancer, disparities exist. Patients from racial and ethnic minority groups are less likely to be referred for testing compared with White patients.[62] In a study of 236 women diagnosed with ovarian cancer from 2012 to 2016, referral rates differed by race with 61% of Caucasian and 40%, 38%, and 33% of Asian, Latina, and Black women, respectively, being referred for genetic testing ($P = .035$),[61] although it is also important to note that closer to 100% of all of these patients should probably have been referred for testing based on current guidelines.[9] This group also found that speaking English ($P<.0001$) and having private or Medicare insurance ($P<.0001$) were significantly associated with higher referral rates.[61] Furthermore, in a study of 6001 patients diagnosed with ovarian cancer from 2013 to 2014, receipt of genetic testing was significantly lower in Black and uninsured patients.[59] Although other studies in patients with ovarian cancer have demonstrated similar findings, these disparities have also been noted in patients who are at higher risk for developing ovarian cancer. For example, once diagnosed with a *BRCA* pathogenic variant, risk-reducing salpingo-oophorectomy rates have been shown to be significantly lower among Black patients compared with Hispanic and non-Hispanic White patients ($P = .025$ and .008, respectively).[58] Taken together, these data suggest that disparities exist along the entire continuum of genetic testing from referral to testing to intervention. Given that select targeted therapies (such as PARP inhibitors) have been shown to vastly improve survival in patients with BRCA-mutated ovarian cancer,[63,64] germline testing in these patients is critical, and disparities at the level of germline genetic testing will undoubtedly affect outcomes.

Although less deadly than ovarian cancer, endometrial cancer is the most common gynecologic malignancy and is one of the only cancers with an increasing incidence in the United States,[34,65] particularly among Black women.[66] Approximately 2% to 5% of endometrial cancers are linked to a heritable cause, mainly genes associated with HNPCC (mismatch repair [MMR] genes *MLH1, MSH2, PMS2, MSH6*, or *EPCAM*)[47] and Cowden syndrome (*PTEN*).[67] In a study of 216 women with uterine cancer, only 13.4% received a genetic referral. Of those referred, 62.1% followed-up for counseling, and 88.9% of those counseled underwent testing.[68] In this study, White patients were more likely to receive a genetic referral compared with Black, Hispanic, Asian, and American Indian/Eskimo patients. Significant factors that favored referral included lower age, lower stage of disease at presentation, and private insurance coverage.[68]

Prostate Cancer

Prostate cancer affects 1 in 7 men in the United States and accounts for 6.7% of male cancer-related deaths.[69] Identifiable genetic variants associated with prostate cancer include *ATM, ATR, BRCA1, BRCA2, BRIP1, CHEK2, FAM175A, GEN1, MRE11A, MSH2, MSH6, NBN, PALB2, PMS2, RAD51C,* and *RAD51D,* and overall genetic variant-related disease accounts for approximately 13.8% of select diagnoses.[70] Notably, VUSs are frequently identified in patients with prostate cancer. In a study of more than 1300 men with prostate cancer who underwent germline testing, these variants were more common in African-American/Canadian (36.6%) and Asian/Pacific Islander (33.3%) men than in Caucasians (21% *P*<.01).[70] In another study of 14,610 patients with prostate cancer, only 667 saw a genetic counselor and 439 underwent genetic testing. Furthermore, this study demonstrated that younger age (<65 year old), having English as one's primary language, having public or private health insurance, and having a family history of prostate cancer were associated with higher rates of testing.[71] This study did not find that race or ethnicity significantly affected rates of referral or testing, although referral and testing rates were quite low overall across all races/ethnicities.[71] As with breast and ovarian cancer, PARP inhibitors have been shown to improve survival outcomes for men with prostate cancer and BRCA1/2 mutations,[72] again highlighting the importance of testing in this population and the need to eliminate disparities in germline genetic testing.

Colorectal Cancer

Colorectal cancer (CRC) is the second most common cause of cancer-related deaths in the United States, and approximately 5% to 10% of CRCs are caused by a heritable pathogenic germline variant.[73] Implicated genes in well-described syndromes include the mismatch repair genes associated with HNPCC (Lynch syndrome; *MLH1, MSH2, MSH6, PMS2,* and *EPCAM*) and FAP (*APC*), with the recessive condition MUTYH-associated polyposis (*MUTYH*), and also with less commonly diagnosed syndromes including Peutz-Jeghers (*STK11*), Cowden (*PTEN*), juvenile polyposis (*BMPR1A*), and other polyposis syndromes (*POLD1, POLE*).[74] In a study of 385 patients with early onset CRC, a majority (76.9%) received immunohistochemistry (IHC) for MMR, with no variance in receipt of IHC by race or ethnicity.[75] However, fewer Black patients were referred for genetic counseling (50.0% vs White patients 54.1% vs Hispanic patients 65.9%, *P* = .02), and fewer Black patients adhered to genetic counseling referral (61.2% vs 81.7% White patients vs 86.2% Hispanic patients, *P*<.01). Of the 141 patients of all races who received genetic testing, 38 (27.0%) had a pathogenic or likely pathogenic variant in a cancer susceptibility gene, and 33 (23.4%) had VUSs, of which 84.8% occurred in racial/ethnic minorities.[75] The literature on testing of *APC* and *MUTYH* genes in non-White and non-Western populations remains limited.[76] However, one study of 6169 patients undergoing genetic sequencing for CRC found that the *APC* mutation rate was higher in Asians, Blacks, and individuals with race reported as "other" compared with Whites (25.2%, 30.9%, 24%, 15.5% respectively; *P*<.0001).[77] However, non-White patients presented with more advanced disease, and thus, the disparity in mutation rates was insignificant after adjusting for polyp burden. In addition, this group found that traditional, restricted testing for the *MUTYH* gene more commonly missed a pathogenic *MUTYH* diagnosis in non-Whites due to allylic variance.[77]

DISCUSSION

Numerous studies have demonstrated the often profound disparities that exist in cancer genetic testing at every step in the process, from identifying patients for testing to referring them for testing to recommending interventions based on the test results. In order to address these failures of our current health care system, significant changes are needed at multiple levels (**Fig. 1**). As a first step, identifying patients could be addressed in several ways. To increase identification, standardized tools are now being incorporated into the electronic medical record, and the push toward risk-based testing is making the use of these tools more imperative. It is now suggested by several groups that a formal risk assessment be done at age 30 years or earlier.[51,78]

Once identified, physicians and other providers need to feel more comfortable with testing, and this can be done by demystifying the testing process, as has been done in the Geisinger health system, in which all PCPs order whole-genome sequencing on their patients.[79] Certifying bodies may also consider deemphasizing extensive pretest counseling, particularly as the number of genes on each panel continues to increase. Furthermore, genetic testing should become part of standard care with reflex referral to genetic counselors and specialists as needed, particularly when pathogenic mutations are diagnosed. As we move forward, one approach could be to target physicians and providers who are in the best position to identify patients for testing of cancer predisposition syndromes and provide educational opportunities to improve their skill set. PCPs in particular may be well positioned to significantly improve patient identification and testing rates, as they typically have more consistent interactions with patients and have developed closer long-term relationships. To improve physicians' knowledge base, several organizations offer educational courses on genetic testing for cancer predisposition syndromes, including City of Hope (https://www.cityofhope.org/education/health-professional-education/cancer-genomics-education-program), the National Consortium of Breast Centers (https://www.breastcare.org/), the American Society of Breast Surgeons (https://www.breastsurgeons.org/), and many others. Free online risk calculators, publications, and national guidelines are also readily available to assist with identifying patients who may meet criteria for testing.[9,31,80] In addition, cascade testing (ie, testing family members of those with known germline mutations) is becoming more common, and it is hoped that integration of cascade testing into primary care practice will expand the number of patients who qualify for and receive genetic testing.

Alternatively, testing could be offered more broadly, thus eliminating some of the confusion around who may or may not qualify for testing. These types of broad testing criteria already exist for select cancers, such as ovarian cancer and pancreatic cancer, neither of which have effective options for population-wide screening. Recently, similar broad-based criteria have been proposed by the ASBrS for all patients with breast cancer to be offered germline genetic testing.[9,11] Furthermore, some have proposed universal population-based testing,[19] as current guidelines are missing a significant number of patients found to harbor pathogenic mutations,[81–83] and the number of studies demonstrating a survival benefit to targeted therapies in BRCA-mutated cancer continues to grow.[50,56,63,72]

Once patients have been appropriately identified for testing, access to testing must also improve; this will likely require a shift in the traditional models of genetic counseling. Given the limited number of genetic counselors available to do counseling,[84] other providers should be encouraged to offer genetic counseling and testing, within the framework of appropriate education and training. Although some have suggested that all genetic testing be performed by genetic counselors, prior studies have shown that test cancellation rates were significantly higher for individuals of African or Latin American ancestry (48.9% and 49.6%, respectively), compared with those of European ancestry (33.9%) when one large national health care insurance payer mandated that testing be done through a genetic counselor specifically, and test positivity rates

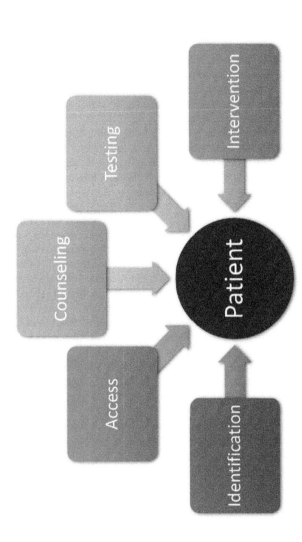

Fig. 1. With the patient as the primary focus, all components of genetic testing need to be addressed to improve disparities in genetic testing.

did not significantly change.[85] Therefore, physicians and other providers will need to help reach all patients who may be eligible for testing; our PCPs in particular may be well suited to help fill this need. However, as with the approach to improving patient identification, provider education will be key, and numerous resources are available.

Another approach to improving access may be to continue to expand telehealth encounters, which have become significantly more common with the recent pandemic. For patients with limited transportation, childcare commitments, restricted availability due to work hours, and/or limited finances, telehealth visits may improve the reach in populations that may otherwise not be able to pursue genetic testing. Telehealth visits for genetic testing have been well studied, and most have shown that it is well received with similar outcomes.[86] Once patients have been tested and a pathogenic mutation identified, numerous resources exist to assist providers with determining the most appropriate management.[9,87] The reasons for disparities in interventions may be more closely related to sociodemographic factors and patient-provider relationships rather than gaps in provider knowledge.

Germline genetic testing offers physicians a potentially life saving tool for identifying and intervening for high-risk individuals. As discussed, historically underrepresented groups are in some cases at an increased risk of carrying a pathogenic variant. Therefore, urgent attention must be paid to these specific populations. Unfortunately, in many cases, genetic testing referral and subsequent care is disproportionately distributed among populations. If correctly used, there is the potential for genetic testing to play a role in decreasing health disparities among individuals of different races and ethnicities.[88] However, if genetic testing continues to revolutionize cancer care while being disproportionately distributed, it also has the potential to widen the existing mortality gap between various racial and ethnic populations in the United States.[89]

FUTURE DIRECTIONS

If current trends continue, the future of oncology will continue to see an expansion of germline genetic testing. The concept of universal testing has been explored for various familial cancer syndromes, with documented survival benefit.[3] Although this approach may be limited by cost and resources, pursuing the best care for all of our patients should remain the priority, regardless of financial constraints.

In addition, if universal genetic testing does become commonplace, the development of large, diverse databases may assist in high-risk patient identification and intervention. As discussed, pathogenic germline variants may carry differing levels of risk in distinct populations. For example, *BARD1* pathogenic/likely pathogenic variants have been strongly associated with estrogen-receptor (ER)-negative breast cancer in Blacks, Hispanics, and Asians but only moderately associated with ER-negative disease in non-Hispanic Whites.[26] The clinical implications of this discrepancy are currently poorly defined, but more robust genomic databases may provide further insight. As this example highlights, creating guidelines based on studies of predominantly White women will undoubtedly affect some of the more vulnerable populations in immeasurable ways. Similar problems have been suggested for breast cancer screening guidelines. These guidelines are shifting toward initiation of screening at an older age based on existing data that largely examined White, nondiverse populations and may disproportionately affect Black populations.[90] Another recurring point of discussion in the studies presented is the high rate of VUSs in minority populations. This discrepancy exists, in large part, due to historical underrepresentation of minority populations in genetic research. Therefore, variants in non-White individuals have not been adequately analyzed, and research in the coming years must focus on this issue and push to reclassify current VUSs. Without testing more diverse populations, clarifying the cancer risk associated with specific genetic variants will remain elusive.

Finally, before the idea of universal genetic testing becomes feasible, medical mistrust must be addressed. In general, public attitudes toward genetic testing have become more positive over time.[91] However, after historical mistreatment in the medical system, minority populations have higher levels of mistrust compared with majority populations.[92] If universal genetic testing becomes a reality, the possibility of widening sociodemographic health gaps based on disproportionate genetic testing uptake remains a looming threat.

SUMMARY

Genetic testing offers providers a potentially life saving tool. However, disparities in receipt of genetic testing have been consistently demonstrated, which is resulting in greater disparities in patient care and outcomes. Therefore, if genetic testing continues to be integrated into routine patient care for those with cancer, continued disproportionate distribution has the potential to widen the existing disparities in outcomes between various racial and ethnic populations.

CLINICS CARE POINTS

- Numerous guidelines exist to determine who should be offered germline genetic testing.
- Genetic testing can be done by several qualified physicians and providers, although genetic counselors remain a valuable resource.
- There are significant disparities noted along the entire continuum of genetic testing, including identification, access, counseling, testing, and intervention.
- Education of providers and patients will be paramount to reducing these disparities, and many resources are available to assist with testing.

DISCLOSURE

K.S. Hughes receives Honoraria from Hologic (surgical implant for radiation planning with breast conservation and wire-free breast biopsy) and Myriad Genetics and has a financial interest in CRA Health (Formerly Hughes RiskApps). CRA Health develops risk assessment models/software with a particular focus on breast cancer and colorectal cancer. K.S. Hughes is a founder and owns equity in the company. K.S. Hughes is the Co-Creator of Ask2Me.Org, which is freely available for clinical use and is licensed for commercial use by the Dana Farber Cancer Institute and the MGH. KH's interests in CRA Health and Ask2Me.Org were reviewed and are managed by Massachusetts General Hospital and Partners Health Care in accordance with their conflict-of-interest policies. JP is the recipient of a research grant from the Color Foundation.

REFERENCES

1. Plichta JK, Griffin M, Thakuria J, et al. What's new in genetic testing for cancer susceptibility? Oncology (Williston Park) 2016;30(9):787–99.
2. Baby's first test: conditions screened by state. Baby's first test. 2020. Available at: https://www.babysfirsttest.org/newborn-screening/states. Accessed June 9, 2021.

3. Samadder NJ, Riegert-Johnson D, Boardman L, et al. Comparison of universal genetic testing vs guideline-directed targeted testing for patients with hereditary cancer syndrome. JAMA Oncol 2021;7(2):230–7.

4. Metcalfe K, Gershman S, Ghadirian P, et al. Contralateral mastectomy and survival after breast cancer in carriers of BRCA1 and BRCA2 mutations: retrospective analysis. BMJ 2014;348:g226.

5. Heemskerk-Gerritsen BAM, Jager A, Koppert LB, et al. Survival after bilateral risk-reducing mastectomy in healthy BRCA1 and BRCA2 mutation carriers. Breast Cancer Res Treat 2019;177(3):723–33.

6. Finch AP, Lubinski J, Møller P, et al. Impact of oophorectomy on cancer incidence and mortality in women with a BRCA1 or BRCA2 mutation. J Clin Oncol 2014; 32(15):1547–53.

7. Møller P, Seppälä T, Bernstein I, et al. Cancer incidence and survival in Lynch syndrome patients receiving colonoscopic and gynaecological surveillance: first report from the prospective Lynch syndrome database. Gut 2017;66(3):464–72.

8. Owens DK, Davidson KW, Krist AH, et al. Risk assessment, genetic counseling, and genetic testing for BRCA-related cancer: US Preventive Services Task Force Recommendation Statement. JAMA 2019;322(7):652–65.

9. Daly MB, Pal T, Berry MP, et al. Genetic/Familial high-risk assessment: breast, Ovarian, and Pancreatic, Version 2.2021, NCCN Clinical Practice Guidelines in Oncology. J Natl Compr Canc Netw 2021;19(1):77–102.

10. Robson ME, Bradbury AR, Arun B, et al. American society of clinical oncology policy statement update: genetic and genomic testing for cancer susceptibility. J Clin Oncol 2015;33(31):3660–7.

11. Manahan ER, Kuerer HM, Sebastian M, et al. Consensus guidelines on genetic' testing for hereditary breast cancer from the American Society of Breast Surgeons. Ann Surg Oncol 2019;26(10):3025–31.

12. Committee opinion No. 693: counseling about genetic testing and communication of genetic test results. Obstet Gynecol 2017;129(4):e96–101.

13. Practice bulletin no. 182 summary: hereditary breast and ovarian cancer syndrome. Obstet Gynecol 2017;130(3):657–9.

14. Giri VN, Hyatt C, Leader A. Cancer screening and genetic testing recommendations for relatives of men undergoing prostate cancer germline testing: implications for practice. J Urol 2020;204(6):1116–8.

15. Syngal S, Brand RE, Church JM, et al. ACG clinical guideline: Genetic testing and management of hereditary gastrointestinal cancer syndromes. Am J Gastroenterol 2015;110(2):223–62 [quiz 263].

16. Pal T, Agnese D, Daly M, et al. Points to consider: is there evidence to support BRCA1/2 and other inherited breast cancer genetic testingfor all breast cancer patients? A statement of the American College of Medical Geneticsand Genomics (ACMG). Genet Med 2020;22(4):681–5.

17. Chapman-Davis E, Zhou ZN, Fields JC, et al. Racial and ethnic disparities in genetic testing at a hereditary breast and ovarian cancer center. J Gen Intern Med 2021;36(1):35–42.

18. Culver JO, Hull JL, Dunne DF, et al. Oncologists' opinions on genetic testing for breast and ovarian cancer. Genet Med 2001;3(2):120–5.

19. King MC, Levy-Lahad E, Lahad A. Population-based screening for BRCA1 and BRCA2: 2014 Lasker Award. JAMA 2014;312(11):1091–2.

20. Shields AE, Burke W, Levy DE. Differential use of available genetic tests among primary care physicians in the United States: results of a national survey. Genet Med 2008;10(6):404–14.

21. Miller FA, Carroll JC, Wilson BJ, et al. The primary care physician role in cancer genetics: a qualitative study of patient experience. Fam Pract 2010;27(5):563–9.
22. ACOG Committee Opinion No. 442: Preconception and prenatal carrier screening for genetic diseases in individuals of Eastern European Jewish descent. Obstet Gynecol 2009;114(4):950.
23. Caswell-Jin JL, Gupta T, Hall E, et al. Racial/ethnic differences in multiple-gene sequencing results for hereditary cancer risk. Genet Med 2018;20(2):234–9.
24. Pal T, Bonner D, Cragun D, et al. A high frequency of BRCA mutations in young black women with breast cancer residing in Florida. Cancer 2015;121(23): 4173–80.
25. Jones T, Trivedi MS, Jiang X, et al. Racial and ethnic differences in BRCA1/2 and multigene panel testing among young breast cancer patients. J Cancer Educ 2021 Jun;36(3):463–9. https://doi.org/10.1007/s13187-019-01646-8.
26. Yadav S, LaDuca H, Polley EC, et al. Racial and ethnic differences in multigene hereditary cancer panel test results for women with breast cancer. J Natl Cancer Inst 2020 Nov 4;djaa167. https://doi.org/10.1093/jnci/djaa167.
27. Lek M, Karczewski KJ, Minikel EV, et al. Analysis of protein-coding genetic variation in 60,706 humans. Nature 2016;536(7616):285–91.
28. Hall MJ, Reid JE, Burbidge LA, et al. BRCA1 and BRCA2 mutations in women of different ethnicities undergoing testing for hereditary breast-ovarian cancer. Cancer 2009;115(10):2222–33.
29. Kurian AW, Li Y, Hamilton AS, et al. Gaps in incorporating germline genetic testing into treatment decision-making for early-stage breast cancer. J Clin Oncol 2017;35(20):2232–9.
30. Eggington JM, Bowles KR, Moyes K, et al. A comprehensive laboratory-based program for classification of variants of uncertain significance in hereditary cancer genes. Clin Genet 2014;86(3):229–37.
31. Plichta JK, Sebastian ML, Smith LA, et al. Germline genetic testing: what the breast surgeon needs to know. Ann Surg Oncol 2019 Jul;26(7):2184–90. https://doi.org/10.1245/s10434-019-07341-8.
32. Institute of Medicine Committee on U, Eliminating R, Ethnic Disparities in Health C. In: Smedley BD, Stith AY, Nelson AR, editors. Unequal treatment: confronting racial and ethnic disparities in health care. Washington (DC): National Academies Press (US) Copyright 2002 by the National Academy of Sciences; 2003.
33. Cancer disparities. NIH: National Cancer Institute; 2020. Available at: https://www.cancer.gov/about-cancer/understanding/disparities. Accessed March 31, 2021.
34. Cancer facts and figures 2020. 2020. Available at: https://www.cancer.org/content/dam/cancer-org/research/cancer-facts-and-statistics/annual-cancer-facts-and-figures/2020/cancer-facts-and-figures-2020.pdf. Accessed March 31, 2021.
35. Morris NS, Field TS, Wagner JL, et al. The association between health literacy and cancer-related attitudes, behaviors, and knowledge. J Health Commun 2013; 18(Suppl 1):223–41.
36. Suther S, Kiros GE. Barriers to the use of genetic testing: a study of racial and ethnic disparities. Genet Med 2009;11(9):655–62.
37. Ozanne EM, O'Connell A, Bouzan C, et al. Bias in the reporting of family history: implications for clinical care. J Genet Couns 2012;21(4):547–56.
38. Kupfer SS, McCaffrey S, Kim KE. Racial and gender disparities in hereditary colorectal cancer risk assessment: the role of family history. J Cancer Educ 2006;21(1 Suppl):S32–6.

39. Genetic Testing Facilities and Cost. BreastCancer.Org. 2016. Available at: https://www.breastcancer.org/symptoms/testing/genetic/facility_cost. Accessed March 31, 2021.
40. Smith CE, Fullerton SM, Dookeran KA, et al. Using genetic technologies to reduce, rather than widen, health disparities. Health Aff (Project Hope) 2016; 35(8):1367–73.
41. Phillips KA, Deverka PA, Hooker GW, et al. Genetic test availability and spending: where are we now? where are we going? Health Aff (Project Hope). 2018;37(5): 710–6.
42. Olaya W, Esquivel P, Wong JH, et al. Disparities in BRCA testing: when insurance coverage is not a barrier. Am J Surg 2009;198(4):562–5.
43. Fogleman AJ, Zahnd WE, Lipka AE, et al. Knowledge, attitudes, and perceived barriers towards genetic testing across three rural Illinois communities. J Community Genet 2019;10(3):417–23.
44. Brown EG, Watts I, Beales ER, et al. Videoconferencing to deliver genetics services: a systematic review of telegenetics in light of the COVID-19 pandemic. Genet Med 2021;1–12.
45. Huang H, Apouey B, Andrews J. Racial and ethnic disparities in awareness of cancer genetic testing among online users: internet use, health knowledge, and socio-demographic correlates. J Consumer Health Internet 2014;18(1): 15–30.
46. Singer E, Antonucci T, Van Hoewyk J. Racial and ethnic variations in knowledge and attitudes about genetic testing. Genet Test 2004;8(1):31–43.
47. Saulsberry K, Terry SF. The need to build trust: a perspective on disparities in genetic testing. Genet Test Mol Biomarkers 2013;17(9):647–8.
48. Siegel RL, Miller KD, Jemal A. Cancer statistics, 2020. CA Cancer J Clin 2020; 70(1):7–30.
49. Yadav S, Couch FJ. Germline genetic testing for breast cancer risk: the past, present, and future. Am Soc Clin Oncol Educ Book 2019;39:61–74.
50. Hu C, Hart SN, Gnanaolivu R, et al. A population-based study of genes previously implicated in breast cancer. N Engl J Med 2021;384(5):440–51.
51. Bevers TB, Helvie MA, Bonaccio E, et al. NCCN guidelines: breast cancer screening and diagnosis (version 1.2020). 2020. Available at: https://www.nccn.org/professionals/physician_gls/pdf/breast-screening.pdf. Accessed December 30, 2020.
52. Alaofi RK, Nassif MO, Al-Hajeili MR. Prophylactic mastectomy for the prevention of breast cancer: Review of the literature. Avicenna J Med 2018;8(3):67–77.
53. Carbine NE, Lostumbo L, Wallace J, et al. Risk-reducing mastectomy for the prevention of primary breast cancer. Cochrane Database Syst Rev 2018;4(4): Cd002748.
54. Robson M, Im SA, Senkus E, et al. Olaparib for metastatic breast cancer in patients with a germline BRCA mutation. N Engl J Med 2017;377(6):523–33.
55. Litton JK, Rugo HS, Ettl J, et al. Talazoparib in patients with advanced breast cancer and a germline BRCA mutation. N Engl J Med 2018;379(8):753–63.
56. Tutt ANJ, Garber JE, Kaufman B, et al. Adjuvant olaparib for patients with BRCA1- or BRCA2-mutated breast cancer. N Engl J Med 2021 Jun 24;384(25):2394–405. https://doi.org/10.1056/NEJMoa2105215.
57. Peterson JM, Pepin A, Thomas R, et al. Racial disparities in breast cancer hereditary risk assessment referrals. J Genet Couns 2020;29(4):587–93.

58. Cragun D, Weidner A, Lewis C, et al. Racial disparities in BRCA testing and cancer risk management across a population-based sample of young breast cancer survivors. Cancer. 2017;123(13):2497–505.
59. Kurian AW, Ward KC, Howlader N, et al. Genetic testing and results in a population-based cohort of breast cancer patients and ovarian cancer patients. J Clin Oncol 2019;37(15):1305–15.
60. Metcalfe KA, Lubinski J, Ghadirian P, et al. Predictors of contralateral prophylactic mastectomy in women with a BRCA1 or BRCA2 mutation: the Hereditary Breast Cancer Clinical Study Group. J Clin Oncol 2008;26(7):1093–7.
61. Hinchcliff EM, Bednar EM, Lu KH, et al. Disparities in gynecologic cancer genetics evaluation. Gynecol Oncol 2019;153(1):184–91.
62. Meyer LA, Anderson ME, Lacour RA, et al. Evaluating women with ovarian cancer for BRCA1 and BRCA2 mutations: missed opportunities. Obstet Gynecol 2010;115(5):945–52.
63. Penson RT, Valencia RV, Cibula D, et al. Olaparib versus nonplatinum chemotherapy in patients with platinum-sensitive relapsed ovarian cancer and a germline BRCA1/2 mutation (SOLO3): a randomized phase III trial. J Clin Oncol 2020;38(11):1164–74.
64. Moore K, Colombo N, Scambia G, et al. Maintenance olaparib in patients with newly diagnosed advanced ovarian cancer. N Engl J Med 2018;379(26):2495–505.
65. Burke WM, Orr J, Leitao M, et al. Endometrial cancer: a review and current management strategies: part I. Gynecol Oncol 2014;134(2):385–92.
66. Henley SJ, Miller JW, Dowling NF, et al. Uterine cancer incidence and mortality — United States, 1999–2016. 2018 Dec 7;67(48):1333–38. https://doi.org/10.15585/mmwr.mm6748a1.
67. Eng C. PTEN: one gene, many syndromes. Hum Mutat 2003;22(3):183–98.
68. Febbraro T, Robison K, Wilbur JS, et al. Adherence patterns to National Comprehensive Cancer Network (NCCN) guidelines for referral to cancer genetic professionals. Gynecol Oncol 2015;138(1):109–14.
69. Howlader N, Noone AM, Krapcho M, et al. SEER cancer statistics review, 1975-2012, National Cancer Institute. Bethesda, MD. Available at: http://seer.cancer.gov/csr/1975_2012/. Accessed March 1, 2021.
70. Kwon DH, Borno HT, Cheng HH, et al. Ethnic disparities among men with prostate cancer undergoing germline testing. Urol Oncol 2020;38(3):80.e81–7.
71. Borno HT, Odisho AY, Gunn CM, et al. Disparities in precision medicine-examining germline genetic counseling and testing patterns among men with prostate cancer. Urol Oncol 2021;39(4). 233.e9–233.e14.
72. de Bono J, Mateo J, Fizazi K, et al. Olaparib for metastatic castration-resistant prostate cancer. N Engl J Med 2020;382(22):2091–102.
73. Siegel RL, Miller KD, Goding Sauer A, et al. Colorectal cancer statistics, 2020. CA Cancer J Clin 2020;70(3):145–64.
74. Giardiello FM, Brensinger JD, Petersen GM. AGA technical review on hereditary colorectal cancer and genetic testing. Gastroenterology 2001;121(1):198–213.
75. Dharwadkar P, Greenan G, Stoffel EM, et al. Racial and ethnic disparities in germline genetic testing of patients with young-onset colorectal cancer. Clin Gastroenterol Hepatol 2020 Dec 24;S1542-3565(20):31721–3. https://doi.org/10.1016/j.cgh.2020.12.025.
76. Hall MJ, Olopade OI. Disparities in genetic testing: thinking outside the BRCA box. J Clin Oncol 2006;24(14):2197–203.

77. Inra JA, Steyerberg EW, Grover S, et al. Racial variation in frequency and phenotypes of APC and MUTYH mutations in 6,169 individuals undergoing genetic testing. Genet Med 2015;17(10):815–21.

78. Monticciolo DL, Newell MS, Moy L, et al. Breast cancer screening in women at higher-than-average risk: recommendations from the ACR. J Am Coll Radiol 2018;15(3 Pt A):408–14.

79. Buchanan AH, Manickam K, Meyer MN, et al. Early cancer diagnoses through BRCA1/2 screening of unselected adult biobank participants. Genet Med 2018; 20(5):554–8.

80. Cintolo-Gonzalez JA, Braun D, Blackford AL, et al. Breast cancer risk models: a comprehensive overview of existing models, validation, and clinical applications. Breast Cancer Res Treat 2017;164(2):263–84.

81. Finch A, Bacopulos S, Rosen B, et al. Preventing ovarian cancer through genetic testing: a population-based study. Clin Genet 2014;86(5):496–9.

82. Beitsch PD, Whitworth PW, Hughes K, et al. Underdiagnosis of hereditary breast cancer: are genetic testing guidelines a tool or an obstacle? J Clin Oncol 2018; 37(6):453–60.

83. Ademuyiwa FO, Salyer P, Ma Y, et al. Assessing the effectiveness of the National Comprehensive Cancer Network genetic testing guidelines in identifying African American breast cancer patients with deleterious genetic mutations. Breast Cancer Res Treat 2019;178(1):151–9.

84. Hoskovec JM, Bennett RL, Carey ME, et al. Projecting the supply and demand for certified genetic counselors: a workforce study. J Genet Couns 2018;27(1): 16–20.

85. Whitworth P, Beitsch P, Arnell C, et al. Impact of payer constraints on access to genetic testing. J Oncol Pract 2017;13(1):e47–56.

86. Raspa M, Moultrie R, Toth D, et al. Barriers and facilitators to genetic service delivery models: scoping review. Interact J Med Res 2021;10(1):e23523.

87. Hughes KS, Parmigiani G, Braun DP. All syndromes known to man evaluator. 2018. Available at: www.ask2me.org. Accessed August 13, 2018.

88. Kashyap MV, Nolan M, Sprouse M, et al. Role of genomics in eliminating health disparities. J Carcinog 2015;14:6.

89. Reid S, Cadiz S, Pal T. Disparities in genetic testing and care among black women with hereditary breast cancer. Curr Breast Cancer Rep 2020;12(3): 125–31.

90. Rebner M, Pai VR. Breast cancer screening recommendations: African American women are at a disadvantage. J Breast Imaging 2020;2(5):416–21.

91. Henneman L, Vermeulen E, van El CG, et al. Public attitudes towards genetic testing revisited: comparing opinions between 2002 and 2010. Eur J Hum Genet 2013;21(8):793–9.

92. Jaiswal J, Halkitis PN. Towards a more inclusive and dynamic understanding of medical mistrust informed by science. Behav Med 2019;45(2):79–85.

93. LaDuca H, Polley EC, Yussuf A, et al. A clinical guide to hereditary cancer panel testing: evaluation of gene-specific cancer associations and sensitivity of genetic testing criteria in a cohort of 165,000 high-risk patients. Genet Med 2020;22(2): 407–15.

94. Couch FJ, Shimelis H, Hu C, et al. Associations between cancer predisposition testing panel genes and breast cancer. JAMA Oncol 2017 Sep 1;3(9):1190–6. https://doi.org/10.1001/jamaoncol.2017.0424.

95. Buys SS, Sandbach JF, Gammon A, et al. A study of over 35,000 women with breast cancer tested with a 25-gene panel of hereditary cancer genes. Cancer 2017;123(10):1721–30.
96. Tung N, Battelli C, Allen B, et al. Frequency of mutations in individuals with breast cancer referred for BRCA1 and BRCA2 testing using next-generation sequencing with a 25-gene panel. Cancer 2015;121(1):25–33.
97. Desmond A, Kurian AW, Gabree M, et al. Clinical actionability of multigene panel testing for hereditary breast and ovarian cancer risk assessment. JAMA Oncol 2015;1(7):943–51.

Moving?

Make sure your subscription moves with you!

To notify us of your new address, find your **Clinics Account Number** (located on your mailing label above your name), and contact customer service at:

Email: journalscustomerservice-usa@elsevier.com

800-654-2452 (subscribers in the U.S. & Canada)
314-447-8871 (subscribers outside of the U.S. & Canada)

Fax number: 314-447-8029

Elsevier Health Sciences Division
Subscription Customer Service
3251 Riverport Lane
Maryland Heights, MO 63043

*To ensure uninterrupted delivery of your subscription, please notify us at least 4 weeks in advance of move.